Digital Mental Health

Digital Mental Health

From Theory to Practice

Edited by

Rob Waller
NHS Lothian

Omer S. Moghraby
West London NHS Trust

Mark Lovell
Tees, Esk and Wear Valleys NHS Foundation Trust

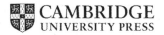
CAMBRIDGE
UNIVERSITY PRESS

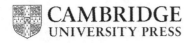

Shaftesbury Road, Cambridge CB2 8EA, United Kingdom

One Liberty Plaza, 20th Floor, New York, NY 10006, USA

477 Williamstown Road, Port Melbourne, VIC 3207, Australia

314–321, 3rd Floor, Plot 3, Splendor Forum, Jasola District Centre,
New Delhi – 110025, India

103 Penang Road, #05–06/07, Visioncrest Commercial, Singapore 238467

Cambridge University Press is part of Cambridge University Press & Assessment,
a department of the University of Cambridge.

We share the University's mission to contribute to society through the pursuit of
education, learning and research at the highest international levels of excellence.

www.cambridge.org
Information on this title: www.cambridge.org/9781009055000

DOI: 10.1017/9781009052023

First published 2023

A catalogue record for this publication is available from the British Library.

Library of Congress Cataloging-in-Publication Data
Names: Waller, Rob, editor. | Moghraby, Omer S., editor. | Lovell, Mark, 1974– editor.
Title: Digital mental health : from theory to practice / Rob Waller, NHS Lothian, Omer S. Moghraby, South London
& Maudsley NHS Foundation Trust, Mark Lovell, Esk and Wear Valleys NHS Foundation Trust.
Description: Cambridge, United Kingdom ; New York, NY : Cambridge University Press, 2023. | Includes
bibliographical references and index.
Identifiers: LCCN 2023024030 (print) | LCCN 2023024031 (ebook) | ISBN 9781009055000 (paperback) |
ISBN 9781009052023 (ebook)
Subjects: LCSH: Internet in psychotherapy. | Medical telematics. | Mental health counseling – Technological
innovations. | Psychotherapy – Technological innovations.
Classification: LCC RC489.I54 D54 2023 (print) | LCC RC489.I54 (ebook) | DDC 616.89/140285–dc23/eng/20230705
LC record available at https://lccn.loc.gov/2023024030
LC ebook record available at https://lccn.loc.gov/2023024031

ISBN 978-1-009-05500-0 Paperback

Contents

Contributors

Paul Bradley
Consultant Psychiatrist and Chief Clinical Information Officer at Hertfordshire Partnership Foundation Trust

Tom Foley
Honorary Senior Clinical Lecturer, Population Health Sciences Institute at Newcastle University; Consultant Child and Adolescent Psychiatrist at the Health Service Executive, Ireland

Fionnbar Lenihan
Consultant Psychiatrist at Defence Forces/ Óglaigh Na hÉireann, Republic of Ireland

Mark Lovell
Consultant Child and Adolescent Intellectual Disability Psychiatrist at Tees, Esk and Wear Valleys NHS Foundation Trust

Donald MacIntyre
Associate Medical Director at NHS 24; Honorary Reader at the University of Edinburgh; Consultant Psychiatrist at NHS Lothian

Omer S. Moghraby
CDIO and Consultant Child and Adolescent Psychiatrist at West London NHS Trust

James Reed
Consultant Forensic Psychiatrist and Chief Clinical Information Officer at Birmingham and Solihull Mental Health NHS Foundation Trust

Hashim Reza
Consultant General Adult Psychiatrist at Oxleas NHS Foundation Trust

Tom Russ
Reader in Old Age Psychiatry, Division of Psychiatry, Centre for Clinical Brain Sciences at the University of Edinburgh; Honorary Consultant Psychiatrist at NHS Lothian; Director, Alzheimer Scotland Dementia Research Centre at the University of Edinburgh; Network Champion, Neuroprogressive and Dementia Network at NHS Research Scotland

Lucy Stirland
Atlantic Fellow for Equity in Brain Health at the Global Brain Health Institute, University of California San Francisco; Honorary Clinical Fellow, Centre for Clinical Brain Sciences, University of Edinburgh

Toral Thomas
Consultant Forensic Psychiatrist and Chief Clinical Information Officer at Norfolk and Suffolk Foundation Trust

Rob Waller
Consultant Psychiatrist, Associate Director of Medical Education and Digital Mental Health Lead at NHS Lothian

Lesa S. Wright
Consultant General Adult Psychiatrist and Chief Technology Officer at Psychiatry-UK LLP

Peter Yellowlees
Alan Stoudemire Endowed Distinguished Professor of Psychiatry, at the University of California–Davis

Introduction

The Changing Landscape of Mental Healthcare

Rob Waller, Mark Lovell and Omer Moghraby

Mental health is a sector that is ripe for digital disruption.
Rebecca Cotton, 2017[1]

Over the past 20 years, we have seen a dramatic shift in how we conduct our daily lives. With digital shopping, ordered items are delivered the same day and communicating is easy with distant family. The years 2020–22 and the global pandemic brought an escalated pace of change, including in healthcare with vaccine appointments booked online.[2] However, the same cannot be said about mental health services where the experiences of both delivering and receiving help lags behind.

This issue was raised by Rebecca Cotton, Director of Policy at the Mental Health Network, in the publication quoted above. If you ask the question 'How much has mental health changed in the last 20 years?', we expect that, like her, your answer will be that it hasn't changed much! Some parts of medicine have, such as how we view radiology images online or how medication is ordered from a GP, but much mental health work is still paper based, delivered in a clinic room and communicated by post.

When home computers became more affordable, several people shared a vision for 'a computer on every desk' – and it could be argued that this has largely been met.[*] There are some important exceptions, but most people now have access to a computer or smartphone. Increasingly, there is access to electronic media in your clinic room; however, it is rudimentary in what we can do with it beyond accessing the Internet or writing and viewing clinical case notes.

A Promised Land?

This book aims to cover the next 10 years, largely looking at what mental health services can reasonably achieve. There may well be a computer in most clinic rooms, but can it do what it needs to do quickly and easily, does the Electronic Health Record (EHR)help or hinder what needs to be done and can service users benefit digitally from other supports and services?

This book is commissioned by the Royal College of Psychiatrists; however, it is aimed at all mental health professionals and other interested parties. The College last wrote a book on *Computers in Psychiatry* 15 years ago and this needs significant updating.[3] There has been an Informatics Committee at the College for many years,[†]

---

[*] Bill Gates, the founder of Microsoft, said this in 1989, but there are earlier mentions.
[†] The Informatics Committee of the Royal College of Psychiatrists meets around three times a year to discuss issues relating to the use of technology, data and information in healthcare, as well as mental

1

which meets termly and has a good representation from across the UK. It is made up of 'clinical informaticians' (digital leaders who are also clinicians) in their own trusts and health boards who are leading the way in digital transformation. Some are at executive level, some are academics and some are front-line clinicians but all want to make sure that the tools are right for the job.

Rebecca Cotton's report makes it clear that technology is the most scalable resource we have and must be seriously integrated in a time of rising demand. Bringing incremental efficiencies to current non-digital pathways will not meet this demand and so innovation needs to be key to how we develop, with much of that innovation being digital in nature.

She also talks about changing expectations in how people access services. For example, they expect 'digital first' and often cannot understand why we still send letters. There will be three main areas of development:

1. Local services – the hardware that every clinician should have easy access to, the systems and processes used, making use of smart and well-designed systems to improve the care delivered.
2. The evidence base – using 'big data' to see the big picture to inform both policy and service development but also real-time clinical decision making.
3. Population mental health – empowering service users and those who support them to self-help, self-determine and prevent mental ill health.

This last area changes so fast in the products that are available and ever-increasing functionality. This includes 'wearables', apps and handheld medical 'devices', which anyone can use to gather increasingly sophisticated information and data about themselves or their families. However, it is not clear who is regulating these, how safe are they, how reliable is the data, who is interpreting and (most importantly) who 'owns' the data?

The next decade is set to be biggest growth area in business and financial investment. Venture capital investment in healthcare technology in the United States doubled from 2019 to the 2020 figure of $14 billion,[4] and a large proportion of that was for mental health ($2.3 billion).[5] Where physical health tech investment has plateaued, mental health tech investment continues to rise, with $5.5 billion spent in 2021. We believe that this investment will drive transformation and innovation in all fields of mental health that is long overdue.

The Changing Landscape

There are many aspects to digital mental health and we will aim to cover most of them. Key topics include technology-enabled care (where computers deliver mental health interventions) and going 'paper-free' to use fully digitised clinical records but ensuring these are fit for purpose. Digitised records then allow for big data (analysing huge datasets as a new way of doing research) and developing technologies like artificial intelligence (with all the ethical questions it throws up). We consider whether we need a new breed of psychiatrists (digital psychiatrists, to help us navigate and change) and the challenge of joining up systems that talk helpfully to our colleagues in social work and beyond. Importantly, we look inwards to the effect technology can have on our own mental health and what digital wellbeing looks like.

health informatics in particular. Members of the Informatics Committee also represent the College at external events and advise on matters of special interest to the Committee. More information is available on their webpage – www.rcpsych.ac.uk/about-us/our-people-and-how-we-make-decisions /other-committees/informatics-committee.

The Landscape Is Rocky

If all this is so wonderful, how come it isn't already happening? Many of us work for the National Health Service (NHS), which is known to move slowly in many areas, but there are some particular rocks that will need to be navigated around.

A major one is that no one has ever done this before. We have had paper for several millennia and in bulk since the printing press was invented in the mid-1400s, but computers have only been in healthcare for several decades. People are concerned about, and have very good questions about, things that they do not understand – the costs as well as the benefits and concerns about information governance.

Service user and professional groups are also concerned about the digital divide,[‡] as whilst most have smart devices and high-speed internet connections, some do not – including some of our more vulnerable service users. Set against this are the benefits we will outline in this book: perhaps they will bring us enough efficiencies that we can more directly help and support those who currently cannot take part.

Who Should Travel This Road?

The purpose of this book is to bring about a change in perspective. We want to highlight the areas ripe for development and support a shift in the mindset of *all* of our workforce that better information, data and digital technology is a core part of mental healthcare.

This book is primarily for mental health professionals. It will aim to provide an overview of the digital mental health landscape to enable you to feel sufficiently empowered to join in, critique and become a driver for change in your local organisation or region. It will also be of relevance to other related groups – patients and service users, other health professionals and those in social care. These are roads that we will be travelling together, keeping each other accountable and sharing what we have learnt.

What Is My Role on the Team?

For some of us, this will be the main focus of our career and the main way in which we impact upon those around us and we have devoted an entire chapter (Chapter 6) to developing digital clinicians, but for most healthcare professionals it will just be a topic of increasing relevance. It is an area that needs us all to engage with, so that it can become a helpful part of our working lives and we can critique it with confidence.

In the Conclusion, we give more detail about how to become involved, but here is a brief list. Some of the terms may make more sense after you have read the book.

- Learn more about the area: most mental health developments, work tools and also conferences will have a digitally focused theme.
- Do a quality improvement or audit project that requires data to be pulled from a Health Information System (such as your EHR).
- Speak to local academics who research big data and assist with a project.
- Submit a 'challenge' to your local innovation team and see how they increasingly can engage with technology firms for a solution.
- Have a coffee with the clinical lead for digital in your organisation – there will be one!

[‡] For information on the digital divide, see https://en.wikipedia.org/wiki/Digital_divide.

- Try video consulting/telepsychiatry – even if just a test call with a friend. Then try it in your job.
- Talk to a colleague in social work or the third sector and explore how your digital systems compare.
- Find a local debate on the ethics of artificial intelligence and go along. Contribute and share!
- Monitor your screen time on your phone or computer and reflect on how this is affecting you. Check which activities you do most and see if changing this helps.
- For members of the Royal College of Psychiatrists – join the Digital Special Interest Group.[§] For members of other organisations, see if they have a similar group.
- Sign up as a member or associate member of a national group or body (e.g. the Faculty of Clinical Informatics,[**] British Computing Society[††] or similar organisations).

The Digital Horizon

Looking back just over 15 years to the College's last book on this topic, you can see that it would be foolish to look too far ahead! However, there are some tensions we can predict and that need to be resolved.

We need to start by using what resources we currently have access to now, which are largely EHRs and electronic prescribing. We then need to develop them and consider putting teams in place to guide this and support their use as staff skills (digital maturity) will vary. We need good frameworks for governance and good clinical leadership here. This also all costs money.

Also, we need to be mindful about how invasive such technology can be – it may invade our personal space more than ever before, with the promise of easier work–life balance typically not realised. Promised cost savings are typically offset by other costs for hardware, software and training. Just because we can use such technology, it does not mean that we should. Paper and pen will still exist and, more importantly, face-to-face human interaction will remain core to our offer of care.

We hope this will be a wise and encouraging journey into digital mental health. Technology should be used as an enabler and to enhance care, and not used just because it exists.

References

1. Cotton, R. *Mental Health and Digital Technology*. Winston Churchill Memorial Trust. 2017. Available at: www .churchillfellowship.org/ideas-experts/idea s-library/mental-health-and-digital-technology (accessed 10 January 2020).

2. Peek, N., Sujan, M., Scott, P. Digital health and care in pandemic times: impact of COVID-19. *BMJ Health Care Inform.* 2020;27(1): e100166.

3. Lenhian, F. *Computers in Psychiatry*. London: Gaskell. 2006.

4. Micca, P., Gisby, S., Chang, C., Shukla, M. *Trends in Healthtech Investment: Funding the Future of Healthcare*. Deloitte Insights. 2021.

[§] Go to www.rcpsych.ac.uk/members/special-interest-groups.
[**] Go to https://facultyofclinicalinformatics.org.uk/payments.
[††] Go to www.bcs.org/membership-and-registrations/become-a-member/.

Available at: www2.deloitte.com/content/ dam/insights/articles/6920_Healthtech- investment-trends/DI_Healthtech- investment-trends.pdf (accessed 6 October 2022).

5. CB Insights. *State of Mental Health Tech 2021 Report*. CB Insights. 2022. Available at: www .cbinsights.com/research/report/mental- health-tech-trends-2021/ (accessed 6 October 2022).

Working with IT Systems
The Benefits and the Challenges

Fionnbar Lenihan

Knowing yourself is the beginning of all wisdom.
Attributed to Aristotle

Introduction

Information flows have been fundamental to life since bacterial chemotaxis allowed our distant ancestors to approach nutrients and flee toxins. More complex organisms have developed ways of sensing the internal as well as external environment. Linked to responsive systems, self-knowledge of this sort is the foundation of the complex homeostasis seen in mammalian bodies.

Organisations and human enterprises are also complex systems at a different level of scale and share fundamental similarities such as a need to sense their environment (both internal and external), process the resulting information and translate it into advantageous actions.

Information technology (IT) should in theory allow this cycle to proceed at a more rapid pace and with less waste. Thus, organisations that adopt IT early and more completely should therefore reap a corresponding improvement in efficiency. That this has not always been the case is a commonplace observation that has become known as the Solow paradox, after the quip by Robert Solow that 'you can see the computer age everywhere but in the productivity statistics'.[1]

In this chapter, we will briefly survey the development of health informatics in the UK, examining some of the more notable examples of the Solow paradox, and try to generalise lessons for the jobbing clinician. We will review current areas of digital deployment in the NHS and look at future prospects, informed by the transformation seen in the recent Covid-19 pandemic.

History and Current State of Health Informatics

Pre-computer

It is said that the founder of medicine, Hippocrates of Kos, insisted on the structured recording of case histories for the benefit of future physicians.[2, 3] The sixteenth-century London Bills of Mortality laid down a list of 81 possible causes of death,[4] anticipating the use of controlled vocabularies, so-called ontologies, or systems of classification, which remain central to health informatics to this day. John Snow (1813–58), anaesthetist and public health physician, famously gathered data and produced what we would now call geospatial data visualisation to allow the location of a cholera outbreak to be determined (the notorious Broad Street pump).[5] Florence Nightingale (1820–1910) too was an accomplished statistician[6] and made pioneering use of data visualisation.[7]

The Electronic Health Record

With the introduction of computers in the 1960s, there was interest in creating systems to help with both clinical and administrative/clerical tasks. It soon became apparent that the 'back office' systems were an easier target for initial efforts. By the 1970s, IT systems were well established in this role in the United States, as well as in the UK in the form of patient administration systems (PAS) that counted and tracked patients but did little more. Lab and radiology systems were also early and relatively unproblematic adoptions both in the United States and UK – the 'C' of CT scans stands for 'computerised' and it quickly became clear that it was easier to make the whole digital file available than to decide which slice of a 3D image to print out on film. The need in the United States for accurate billing and coding drove a need for IT systems to support these US-specific initiatives such as the move to health maintenance organisations (HMO) and managed care in the 1980s. This was mirrored in the UK by the introduction of Resource Management Initiative (RMI)/ Casemix systems to support the then-current political objectives about tracking and costing healthcare inputs and outputs.

Initial interest in creating artificial intelligence (AI) diagnostic systems (expert systems such as MYCIN and INTERNIST-I) did not seem to result in their widespread adoption outside academia.[8] More modest initiatives such as Medline in 1965 aimed to support, not supplant, expert decision making with access to current evidence and, more recently, so-called decision support tools.

Starting from small beginnings as early as 1975, UK primary care transformed from a paper-based to a computerised system, meaning that there has been a comprehensive Electronic Health Record (EHR) at the point of care for some years now.[*] There are reliable mechanisms for transfer of records within primary care between practices when a patient moves and also in summary form to secondary care on referral or admission (the Summary Care Record). This is a little-known success story of UK health informatics and this contrast with the more varied history of secondary care IT deserves some examination.[9]

General practitioners (GPs) are, in effect, small business owners and they have a personal investment in their workflows and processes that may be lacking in secondary care. The GP workforce contained many enthusiastic early adopters of EHRs who, in some cases, wrote the software they used. This intimate involvement of domain specialists was lacking in secondary care and has highlighted a need for a hybrid clinician–informatician role (described in more detail in Chapter 6). There were also several supportive policy and incentive frameworks that helped drive primary care to adopt EHRs,[10] including paying GPs a premium if they were able to deliver screening interventions to certain proportions of their caseload.

In the United States, concern over iatrogenic harm was an important driver of IT adoption under the reasonable assumption that IT systems could be used to reduce

---

[*] Various terms exist for this – we have gone with 'Electronic Health Record' or EHR. Related terms are Electronic Patient Record, Digital Health Record or Electronic Notes. These are discussed in more detail in Chapter 3.

human error. However, the potential for IT systems to compromise patient privacy and confidentiality were identified early on and helped drive the 1996 US Health Insurance Portability and Accountability Act (HIPAA) requirements of confidentiality and legibility.[3] IT systems were (and are) often seen as a way of squaring the circle of maintaining or improving quality in an era of increasing demand and reduced funding. Therefore, it is perhaps no surprise that the Health Information Technology for Economic and Clinical Health (HITECH) Act of 2009 was part of the US response to the global financial crisis of 2008 that mandated,[3] and more importantly funded (to the value of $30 billion),[11] the widespread adoption of EHRs in the United States. The return on this investment was an increase in EHR use from 10% to 75% across a wide range of healthcare providers from small clinics to large hospitals.

The lag between primary and secondary care in the adoption of IT (as early as 1991, more than 60% of UK GP practices had adopted EHRs[12]) continued to concern governments in the UK and a range of initiatives and strategies were tried. The New Labour administration in the late 1990s saw a transformative potential in the creation of a single unified national EHR, leading to the National Program for IT (NPfIT) in 2002,[13] a major initiative that will be examined in the National Program for IT section.

The devolved administration in Scotland, along with Wales and Northern Ireland, chose to remain separate from this. In Scotland, a more gradualist approach was taken which involved tolerating a mix of systems whilst aiming to gradually integrate this over time using portal systems and gateways.

In the European Union (EU), the Commission's Communication on the 'digital transformation of health and care' of April 2018 laid out the EU strategy on health informatics.[14] It consists of three pillars covering secure data access and information sharing across the EU, the sharing of information to improve individual and collective healthcare through research and strengthening citizen empowerment through digital services.

Telepsychiatry (Also Known as Video Consultations)

Telepsychiatry is the use of electronic communication and information technologies to provide or support mental healthcare at a distance.[15] As a relatively 'hands-off' speciality, it is a natural candidate for remote delivery and the first experiments along these lines started in the 1950s when the Nebraska Psychiatric Institute delivered interventions over an early (analogue) videoconferencing link.[16] An important point is that the interventions included not just doctor–patient consultations but also professional–professional meetings and teaching sessions. This shows the importance of thinking laterally.

In the 1970s, a regular psychiatry clinic was delivered to Logan Airport health clinic by remote means.[16] Australia, too, was an early adopter of telepsychiatry, perhaps due to that continent's large geography.[17] Peter Yellowlees and others did important work demonstrating the value of telepsychiatry, including with underserved groups such as Indigenous Australians, who might not have seemed natural candidates for telepsychiatry.[18] He is the author of Chapter 7 in this book, where he explores telepsychiatry in much more detail.

The common perception remained, however, that telepsychiatry was 'second best' to face-to-face consultation and best suited to particular environments such as Australia or the polar regions. The Covid-19 pandemic has provided an enormous impetus to telepsychiatry with a very rapid pivot to remote consultations. The results of this natural experiment are awaited with interest. In the interim it behoves practitioners to familiarise themselves with formal good practice guidelines for their speciality and their jurisdiction. The Irish coalition group Mental Health Reform have helpfully produced a document summarising European, Irish, UK and US guidance.[19]

Box 1.1 details the chapter author's personal experience with setting up a telepsychiatry service in a regional mental health unit.

E-Learning

Just as e-commerce was prefigured by catalogue shopping; it could be argued that e-learning was foreshadowed by correspondence courses,[21] or the Open University,[22] which was

---

Box 1.1 Personal experience with telepsychiatry

Telepsychiatry can be provided with good-quality video and audio and can cover almost all aspects of a mental health consultation, especially if there is support for the service user on hand.

In 2008–9, we were able to obtain an obsolete videoconferencing unit that was being discarded by the management suite. We later took advantage of a Scottish government initiative to have a second unit bought for us.

We initially envisaged 'telepsychiatry' as involving only doctor–patient contact. In 2017, however, the long-term sick leave of a colleague required us to find ways of getting more out of our reduced medical workforce. We therefore introduced a system of 'virtual clinics' where consultants provided support and advice to prison-based senior nurses (most with pre-scriber training). This was, despite the modest scope of the initiative, very popular and helped greatly reduce referrals to psychiatry from prison and the impact of our absent colleague. We ended the period of sick leave with a shorter waiting list than when we started!

The recent pandemic situation led to an abrupt adoption of doctor–patient telepsychiatry by many psychiatrists. The chapter author's main experience of this is in his current role as a military psychiatrist in the Republic of Ireland and is generally positive. Military facilities are often very widely scattered and travel between them was more problematic with pandemic restrictions. The experience of telepsychiatry consultations in the pandemic needed to be compared not with 'normal' face-to-face interactions but with masked and socially distanced ones, and in this comparison they came out as superior. The main concern was if the person being examined was significantly distressed, but this was addressed by making sure they had support with them at their end.

In terms of practice points, the stability of the connection is very important. Sound quality is critical, perhaps more than video quality (beyond a certain minimum). It is important to consider the IT skills of the population you are serving, as well as their access to IT devices, high-speed broadband or even a private area in their home from which to connect. This issue came up in our work in the prisons, with remote units being vandalised or tampered with. Yellowlees even suggested the use of the patient's car as a private secure space,[20] particularly when parked close enough to the home to get a Wi-Fi signal, and this indeed has proved useful on occasions.

One model that has proved successful is a hybrid one where a remote consultation supports a local practitioner such as a specialist nurse or a primary care practitioner who is physically present with the patient. This may represent a very workable middle point for many mental health consultations following the lifting of pandemic restrictions

Confidentiality and consent are particularly important in remote consultations and adherence to national/local policies and best practice guidelines as well as scrupulous documentation are highly recommended.

founded in 1969. With the widespread availability of networked home computers, e-learning moved onto the Internet or internal corporate intranets.

Much like telepsychiatry, it is important to look at e-learning in a lateral way as encompassing a range of approaches from standalone 'packages' that need to be worked through to complex online environments which shape and facilitate educational interactions.

There is no learning currently that is not 'e' to some degree. Most face-to-face teaching involves scheduling, the distribution of materials by email and is often supported by an online resource. It is also the case that the open Internet contains a wide range of educational material, often curated and of high quality, such as Coursera or the Open University.[23] However, there are excellent reasons to create a 'walled garden' online for students, particularly for highly regulated careers such as medicine, so virtual learning environments (VLEs) are required. Blackboard[24] and Moodle[25] are examples of this kind of software. Some of these offerings are open source, some commercial. Open source offers reassurances around the issue of interoperability and vendor lock-in (being tied to an expensive system purchased some time ago) that has parallels in healthcare IT.

The functionality of VLEs varies but typically includes support for administrative functions such as access control, staff contact lists, syllabi, timetables, scheduling and reading lists. There are typically libraries for content such as lectures, presentations and study notes. Increasingly, learning is seen as an active process of engagement rather than passive rote learning, so features such as bulletin boards, chat and collaborative editing environments are included. Tests and quizzes can be built into a VLE, including for student feedback. In work-based VLEs such as those used by many healthcare organisations for mandatory training modules, a passing grade on these tests can provide confirmation of adherence to mandatory training. Finally, the creation of persistent records of learning, such as portfolios, may support assessment and regulatory needs.[26]

Separate but connected to VLEs is the topic of simulation. Simulations in medical training can be quite low-tech, such as banana-skin suturing, or as high-tech as robotic patients for intubation and resuscitation. These manual skills are relatively rarely needed in mental health settings but are important to acquire, so experience of a medical emergency in a simulated setting can be valuable learning. Simpler, narration-based tools can be used to create simulations of clinical situations in psychiatry without the hardware or programming overheads of complex graphics. One interesting option is the work by O'Shea, Lenihan and Semple using an interactive fiction design tool called Twine to create branching clinical scenarios with if/then logic and scores.[27]

A recurring theme in this chapter is the importance of focusing on the end goal, not the technology used to achieve it, and how the introduction of IT should not be primarily for reasons of convenience or finance. These lessons apply to e-learning as much as to EHRs or telepsychiatry.

There are technical and legal issues around creating content for online learning, which can be minimised by using the tools, personnel and resources provided by your institution. There are also issues relating to file size and format that may inconvenience your users. Be particularly careful not to include the copyrighted material of others without appropriate permissions. Even when material may be freely reused, there remains the scholarly duty of appropriate recognition and attribution. Licensing affects your own creative work too. Depending on local institutional arrangements you may, or may not, be free to distribute your work online. Even if you favour the most 'generous' sharing policy, it may still be wise to exert some form of control using Creative Commons tools.[28]

There are ethical and (depending on your jurisdiction) legal requirements to ensure that your teaching materials and tools are accessible to a neurodiverse student population and to students with other disabilities such as visual impairments. Most of these principles represent common-sense good design in any case, such as unique titles for slides, good contrast and minimal visual clutter on slides. A useful summary is provided by the 'Full Fabric' blog.[29]

Past Failures

This is a book about the future of digital mental health, but we do need to look at and learn from the past or we will be doomed to repeat its mistakes.[†]

Problems with Public Sector IT Procurement

Whilst public sector IT procurement failures attract much attention, it is probably worth noting at the outset that there may be a publication bias at work as private corporations do not have the same requirements for transparency and accountability,[30] and may thus be better placed to quietly bury their failures. A *Computerworld* article from early 2020 lists some recent examples from the private sector.[31]

Other governments and organisations are however not immune to these difficulties. According to a 2003 report, in the period between 2003 and 2012, only a distinct minority of large US IT projects were successful.[32]

Problems with Electronic Health Records

In the United States, EHR systems typically emerged as add-ons to existing customer billing/finance systems and were not optimised for clinical workflows; it is no surprise therefore that EHR software was cited as a cause in more than 50% of US cases of physician burnout. They have been accused of making it too easy for third parties to request 'just one more' item of information, leading physicians and other healthcare professionals to become data-entry clerks rather than health professionals. They also lead to perverse incentives, with high percentages of patients having enough symptoms to count as complex because physicians get paid more for complex cases. The story of EHR development in the United States is told by Bob Wachter in his light-hearted book *The Digital Doctor*.[33]

One UK example is the Casemix Information Systems and Resource Management Initiative (CMIS/RMI). These were programs introduced in the mid-1980s which were intended to have a strategic and integrative function, sitting in the centre of existing clinical and managerial IT systems. The goal was to have the ability to establish the notional costs of each episode of patient care, which in aggregate created the 'casemix' of the hospital. Clinical activity (consultations, investigations, etc.) were recorded along with financial data and used to compare clinical and financial performance with a standard or idealised case. The lack of perceived clinical benefit and buy-in contributed to the eventual failure of the program, though elements have been subsumed into later systems.

[†] Attributed to Gregory Santayana (1863–1952).

The National Program for IT

Background

The National Program for IT (NPfIT) ran between 2002 and 2011. During its period of operation, it is reported to have cost £12.4 billion. Connecting for Health (CfH) was the arm's-length body charged with delivering NPfIT and for most of its active existence (until 2008) it was led by Richard Granger, a former civil servant and management consultant with experience in large-scale IT procurement.

It is important to understand that, whilst the end goal of the initiative was to deliver a comprehensive national EHR, this involved creating several foundation components, including the network itself, electronic mail, the 'spine', a range of national applications like 'Choose and Book', as well as the picture archiving and communication system (PACS). It was a huge task.

The approach taken was to divide England into five geographical 'clusters' in each of which a local service provider was contracted to deliver the agreed product as a local monopoly. Steep financial penalties were agreed for non-performance of the contracts. Under these conditions, procurement proceeded quickly, and this was positively commented on. Over time, however, this adversarial approach drained goodwill from the enterprise and once technical problems and delays emerged, inevitable in a project of this size and complexity, relationships soured. There was a high turnover of experienced staff with consequent loss of corporate knowledge. Key deadlines were missed and supplied systems were sometimes not sufficiently reliable. There were complaints that NHS staff had not been engaged as stakeholders, together with conflict with the public and professional bodies about the consent model for sharing information between different systems.

By 2009, NPfIT had not come close to delivering the integrated national EHR that had been envisaged, and following criticism from the Public Accounts Committee in January 2009, the incoming coalition government terminated the project in 2011.

Successes

It is important to mention the significant successes from this program. These include important infrastructure such as the improved NHS network with a central 'spine' for storing and exchanging information, an electronic prescribing system, the PACS image system, the Summary Care Record, the NHS mail staff email system and the Choose and Book appointment system. These are still in use today.

Failures

The Wachter report of 2016 identified a number of factors for the failure of NPfIT.[34] The most basic, according to the report and other authors, such as Dolfing,[35] Coiera[36] and Robertson and colleagues,[37] was simply scale. There was no 'plan B', no ability to gracefully degrade to a down-scoped version of the program. Another key issue according to the report and other sources was the ambitious, perhaps unrealistic, timetable. Other problems included the excessively centralised approach to contracting and procurement and the excessively confrontational nature of these processes, which served to alienate the suppliers and lead to them charging heavily for modifications to poorly written specifications.

This led to problems downstream where professional groups and other stakeholders delayed progress and where vague specifications led to legal disputes and unclear project scope. Pressure of time also contributed to a lack of testing with resulting quality control issues, delays and the reliability issues mentioned above.

Wachter and others noted the lack of clinical engagement with the project and highlighted that this needed to be something that happens at the beginning of a project, not the end. A lack of expertise, both in 'pure' IT skills and also in the critical IT/clinician crossover area, was identified.

Lessons Learned

The large-scale strategic learnings from NPfIT are representative of other large-scale procurements. These include the need to recognise the complexity of the problem and the need for 'adaptive change' (where the whole system needs to change as well as the IT system). Also, due to the lag between implementation and realisation of benefits, organisations need to respect this and understand that the return on investment may not be financial. Crucially, technical support and a willingness to adjust the solution should extend past the implementation, through the inevitable teething problems and on through the adaptive change process.

Motives are important. Digitisation/computerisation should happen for clinical reasons, not IT, financial or managerial reasons. The clinical workforce needs to *believe* this (that they are not having a management system foisted on them) and so be on board for the inevitable pain and disruption this kind of adaptive change involves. There needs to be efforts made to upskill the workforce and to foster the hybrid clinician/informatician role as the necessary process re-engineering involved in adaptive change requires deep domain knowledge combined with an understanding of the technology. Wachter recommended the creation of Chief Clinical Information Officers (CCIOs) at both local and national levels to support this.

Wachter warned against dramatic crash programmes. He recommended sensitivity to the level of readiness of the organisation with different combinations of incentives and regulation over time for organisations in order to bring them all to a sufficient position of 'digital maturity'.

Also, Wachter cautioned about over-generalising the lessons of NPfIT and completely rejecting centralisation. He recommended a balance between centralisation and devolved implementation. Large-scale EHR systems have enormous potential for healthcare research and public health so there needs to be balance in the area of privacy and also a clear external regulatory framework and mechanisms to support information interchange.

More specific learnings include the importance of interoperability and the need to establish this at the outset. Without this, the risk of 'vendor lock', dependence on a single supplier, is too high. Interoperability and open standards also foster an ecosystem of innovation. Interoperability can mean the centralised mandating of *how* systems share information but allow different parts of the system to use different products that suit their particular needs.

Complexity can be tamed by modularisation and staging of projects and Wachter recommended aiming for initial 'quick wins' to build momentum and enhance morale. He also touched on user engagement and the usability of the user interface/user experience (UI/UX) at the design stage, informed by an understanding of the cognitive demands on clinicians. Gaining this understanding will require ethnographic approaches to UI/UX design. This is covered more in Chapter 4 on EHRs and digital note keeping.

The good news is that implementing an EHR can be done better and Box 1.2 contains the author's personal experience with a full EHR transition which, whilst not perfect, did illustrate some of the points above.

In addition to all the useful points listed in Box 1.2, our experience would suggest that developments have a natural time and pace and that there is no point forcing a development before this natural time. The corollary to this is the importance of recognising and taking advantage of the right time when it comes. Crises often drive developments, and notwithstanding the difficulties of crash projects, it can be a good idea to have draft plans drawn up and ready for implementation when the right moment arrives.

Wachter was undoubtedly correct when he highlighted the importance of having health professionals involved in IT projects. However, IT professionals often fail to understand just how variegated and diverse modern healthcare professions are and may regard a generic clinician such as a surgeon a satisfactory representative of all clinical professionals and specialties. Hence it needs to be clinicians *plural* involved and not just one lone worker.

Box 1.2 Personal experience with EHR transition

The author's experience stems from working in a regional medium secure unit in Scotland. This unit, opening in 2000, presciently ordered an early version of an EHR from a UK supplier so that it was operating in a paperless/paper-light mode from the outset. Over time, the application proved popular and useful. The EHR system was not without its flaws but professionals from all disciplines became deeply familiar with it and learned to work around many of these. There had, however, been little planning around long-term support, succession or data portability.

By 2016, withdrawal of support by Microsoft for their older operating systems, increasing worries about compatibility going forward, along with obsolescence of the EHR software itself, were causing concern. Around this time, the wider organisation's mental health services were in the process of transitioning to a very large and widely deployed EHR system used by the physical health part of the organisation. A decision was made to volunteer the medium secure unit to be an early adopter for mental health of the new EHR.

This was not a universally popular decision. The rationale and need for the transition were not apparent to everyone and perhaps had not been communicated effectively. The new EHR, by virtue of being used across multiple secondary care settings, was not tuned to any one specialty and did not support some beloved features despite attempts to make compensatory modifications. The interface could also be best described as 'functional'. However, staff were trained and on-site support with clinical leadership was available.

There were, however, some major advantages. As a critical part of NHS Lothian's infrastructure, we could be confident that the whole organisation would support our EHR going forward rather than the responsibility resting with a small forensic clinic. Similarly, the financial costs lay with the organisation as a whole rather than a small part of it. Doctors in training and other short-term staff could be quickly effective as it was the same EHR they were used to using elsewhere. The new system gave us access to medical and surgical notes, outpatient appointments and to radiology and laboratory results. Our patients being looked after in general medical/surgical settings could get better care due to there being joined-up record keeping. Perhaps most importantly for these patients with high needs and risks, all records were in one place, making it less likely that a vital piece of information was missed when compiling risk assessments or other documents.

Current and Near-Future Issues

UK Structures

In the UK, the Wachter report called for a '5-year-forward view' with ubiquitous EHRs and e-prescribing.[34] There was a recognition of the varying degrees of digital maturity across England and Wales and a focus on interoperability and personalised healthcare.

In 2019, NHSX was created to coordinate IT delivery across health and social care across England and Wales. It has had a strategic role, setting policy and standards with actual implementation being commissioned by NHS Digital. In 2022, it was integrated into the NHS Transformation Directorate but progress had been made with a more helpful level of centralisation, the ongoing creation of regional integrated care services with a requirement to share data digitally across health and social care and better clarity of 'what good looks like' and 'who pays for what'.[38]

National structures will undoubtedly continue to evolve. Digital departments have definitely arrived – the challenge now is to embed it as 'business as usual' so we don't need the sub-focus of digital at all.

Pandemic Response

At the time of writing (Spring 2022), we are two years into the global Covid-19 pandemic but there are signs of more normality returning. However, ongoing periodic waves of infections including the annual winter bed crisis mean that we need to continue to implement the lessons learned during this stressful time.

Telepsychiatry and tele-mental health therefore will be an obvious IT application for the immediate future. Ease of use will be improved, as will integration with EHR systems. We will have to give more thought to the 'distal', or patient, end of the telepsychiatry link with ruggedised or tamperproof systems for certain environments. The status of telepsychiatric assessments with respect to statutory processes such as detention will need to be clarified, having already been challenged in court. It is likely that telepsychiatry will be part of a spectrum, or menu, of options in the post-pandemic situation, particularly for military services or for remote areas or areas where access is difficult (e.g. prisons, ships).

The adoption of EHRs is likely to accelerate also due to the pandemic because of their ability to support remote working, easier integration with telepsychiatry, reduction in travel and thus reduced movement of potential infected persons and fomites.

Resilience and Disaster Management

One of the lessons of the pandemic is, or ought to be, an increased sense of the vulnerability of our globally interconnected world. Going forward, more will be asked of healthcare IT in terms of resilience to, for example, power outages, network problems, cyberattacks and extreme weather events. In addition, IT systems will be expected to display 'graceful degradation' under these conditions with backups available rather than abrupt collapse. Ensuring this happens will become an important part of the specification process.

There are increasing concerns regarding foreign suppliers for key items of infrastructure including important public sector IT hardware and software. This is on the basis of supply chain reliability but also due to security concerns, as we saw with recent disputes over the Chinese company Huawei and 5G networks. For example, both the United States and the EU are 'onshoring' microprocessor production. Going forward, bidding for strategic IT investments such as large public healthcare systems may be confined to trusted partner companies based in friendly or allied nations. Shrinking the pool of available suppliers will inevitably lead to reductions in choice and increases in cost. On a more positive note, closer working relationships with a small number of trusted partners may help reduce the adversarial procurement practices identified as a factor in the NPfIT debacle.

Mobility and Remote Access

It has been noted that the interposition of a computer screen between clinician and patient can significantly degrade the quality of clinical interactions and contribute to clinician burnout. Breaking the umbilical cord and allowing the EHR to be read to, and written from, on a more flexible, paper-like device has long been of interest to IT companies. Long before the iPad launched in 2010, Microsoft pushed the concept of the 'tablet PC' for many lonely years with a clear emphasis on so-called 'vertical' markets including healthcare. It may have been that, in classic chicken and egg fashion, EHRs were not yet ubiquitous enough to justify the use of expensive (as they were then) specialist tablet hardware. The profusion of tablet-style devices since then and the widespread use of EHR systems perhaps makes this option worth revisiting. A flat tablet-style device using well-designed menus and dropdowns, along with handwriting and voice recognition, could allow real-time access to EHR systems along with preserved patient rapport. Such a device, along with a lightweight portable keyboard and cellular networking, could act as an EHR terminal, a telepsychiatry workstation and a portable office and might be all the IT infrastructure many mobile mental health workers will need.

Carbon Footprint

Environmental concerns have taken a back seat in global conversations over the last year, but the underlying problems have not gone away. There are simple and direct environmental advantages of many health informatic developments, including reductions in travel time and the transport and storage of physical records, both energy-consuming activities.

Data centres, however, are a major consumer of energy and electronic hardware raises important environmental questions from both raw material mining and waste disposal perspectives. Recent initiatives such as mandatory energy efficiency, new designs for data centres and 'right to repair' laws may help tilt the balance towards the positive.

It is likely that those planning the introduction of ambitious IT projects will have to include in their business cases a detailed accounting of these costs and benefits.

Manpower Issues

Specialisation and division of labour have long been seen as an important driver of improved quality and reduced costs.[39] However, if specialist services see a high number of particular conditions or carry out a high number of specific procedures to get their better outcomes, it is difficult to see how this increasing division of work can be safely coordinated without tools like shared EHRs and computer-assisted workflows.

An ageing population exacerbates this problem with more episodes of care, spread over more specialties and sites, more professionals involved and more medications being prescribed. Managing this 'multimorbidity' will be very difficult without the tools described in this book. As well as being more specialised, the healthcare workforce is becoming more diverse and working shorter hours, so systems will be designed to support handovers, briefings, huddles and the rapid acquisition of situational awareness.

There are shortages in several categories of healthcare worker and, for some underserved areas and populations, telepsychiatry, e-learning and decision support systems will be needed to augment the limited professional workforce. Integrating these developments in a safe and defensible way will be a major challenge for the years to come.

Future Prospects

The aphorism that 'it is difficult to make predictions, particularly about the future' has been attributed to various sages. Regardless of the provenance, however, it remains a good guide when making predictions about the future. The author edited a book some years ago which was bold enough to include a list of predictions.[40] The reader may wish to consult these and compare them with today's reality before deciding how much credence to give to the further prognostications below!

Infrastructure

It seems a safe place to start to predict that EHR systems will become universal with paper-based records only used for retrospective case review. These will increasingly be accessed by mobile devices in a range of form factors rather than fixed terminals.

A range of factors are pushing towards ubiquitous, wide-area, high-speed mobile networking to the point that many people may have only a 'mobile' connection at home and the current distinction between local Wi-Fi and wide-area 3G/4G/5G networks will blur.

With mass production, and economies of scale, cameras and sensors are now cheap and almost disposable. Cost pressures, along with liability and governance issues, will act as a driver for these to be incorporated into care environments, for example, as sensors for non-contact respiration monitoring in seclusion rooms, medication compliance sensors on pill boxes, or for detecting falls in the elderly. Many of these sensors will feed their data directly into EHR systems, reducing the need for manual transcription but increasing the volume of raw data that clinicians will have to contend with. There will be complex ethical, privacy, legal and clinical trade-offs to navigate.

Not all monitoring will be non-consensual or covert. One of the genuinely novel and unexpected trends since our book has been the degree to which people are willing to monitor themselves and to give up large volumes of personal data for minimal or no reward.[40] We are all familiar with the patient who brings along voluminous diaries and other writings to be reviewed in a finite appointment time. The proliferation of mood diary apps, wearable devices, trackers and home diagnostic systems will increase this 'co-creation' of medical information and our systems will need to learn to store, and render meaningful, these new information sources.

Analysis

Proceeding from the preceding point, these large datasets (big data) will need automated processing and analysis if they are to generate meaning. We can envisage research and audit moving from something that happens retrospectively to something that happens continuously in real time with tight loops between practice and evaluation.

At the time of writing, AI is going through one of the regular peaks of hype to which it is prone.[41] It is, of course, not a singular thing and the AI term encompasses several different approaches. Many of these approaches are not algorithmic or rule based but use neural networks, statistical models or genetic algorithms. These tools are not based on explicit representation of the problem domain or the solution and, even if accurate, are not transparent or explainable. This can pose problems when the AI generates categories which violate social norms,[42] or when decision-making transparency is legally required. 'Explainable' AI is at an early stage but would seem like an important initiative.[43] Chapters 4 and 5 of this book focus on big data and AI along with the associated ethical concerns.

Standards and Security

We have seen above how interoperability of EHR systems is already important and will become only more so if we are to avoid vendor lock-in and facilitate modularisation. The best way to achieve durable and resilient interoperability is for vendors to ensure that their systems adhere to open, published standards. Proprietary standards, which can be manipulated by market players, are to be avoided if possible.

Another major issue will be security. The concept of 'hybrid warfare' blurs the state/non-state actor distinction by incorporating the use of deniable assets to disrupt adversary IT systems. The migration of critical national infrastructure like EHR systems online opens up the possibility of mass casualties from such attacks. We saw a ransomware attack on NHS

Table 1.1 Key lessons – risks and controls in health IT projects

Risks	Controls
Failure to appreciate complexity, scale and interrelatedness of the proposed project.	Consider breaking project down into more manageable sub-projects, modules or stages.
Failure to achieve buy-in from end users and other stakeholders.	Stakeholder engagement.
Failure to change the skill mix of users.	Training and recruitment.
Underbudgeting.	Realistic budgeting including implementation, training and customisation costs.
Adversarial procurement processes leading to loss of good will.	Better management of supplier relationships.
Scope creep – the addition of new features mid-project.	Discipline and management of stakeholders. Ability to say no.
Failure to re-engineer workflows to suit the new IT system.	Don't 'put lipstick on a pig', that is, blindly replicate an old, suboptimal or purely paper-based process in new software.

systems (Wannacry) in 2017 and this will not be the last. There may be a need for binding international agreements making attacks on health infrastructure a war crime in the same way as attacks on dams. In the interim, end users and the public will need to accept significant convenience trade-offs in order to maintain security.

Conclusions

The scope of this chapter was broad and could easily have justified an entire book of its own. I hope, however, that it, and the additional resources referenced, will set the scene for some of the more specialist chapters that follow and allow the reader to ask some sensible initial questions if they are asked to become involved in a digital project. Some of the most key lessons of the NPfIT, from both Wachter and others, are summarised in Table 1.1.

References

1. Krishnan, M., Mischke, J., Remes, J. Is the Solow Paradox back? *McKinsey Quarterly*, 4 June 2018. Available at: www.mckinsey.com/capabilities/mckinsey-digital/our-insights/is-the-solow-paradox-back#/ (accessed 20 June 2023).

2. Nissen, T., Wynn, R. The history of the case report: a selective review. *JRSM Open*. 2014;5(4): 205427041452341. https://doi.org/10.1177/2054270414523410.

3. McLean, K. Intro to history of health informatics. *YouTube*. 26 January 2013. Available at: www.youtube.com/watch?v=AzLy58dhsXc (accessed 8 January 2022).

4. Morabia, A. Observations made upon the Bills of Mortality. *BMJ*. 2013;346: e8640. https://doi.org/10.1136/bmj.e8640.

5. Choi, B. C. The past, present, and future of public health surveillance. *Scientifica*. 2012: 1–26. https://doi.org/10.6064/2012/875253

6. Neuhauser, D. Florence Nightingale gets no respect: as a statistician that is. *Qual. Saf. Health Care*. 2003;12(4): 317. https://doi.org/10.1136/qhc.12.4.317.

7. Gupta, S. Florence Nightingale understood the power of visualizing science. *Science News*. 13 May 2020. Available at: www.sciencenews.org/article/florence-nightingale-birthday-power-visualizing-science (accessed 8 January 2022).

8. Clinfowiki. Medical informatics history. *Clinfowiki*. 2011. Available at: www.clinfowiki.org/wiki/index.php/Medical_in formatics_history (accessed 8 January 2022).

9. Benson, T. Why general practitioners use computers and hospital doctors do not – part 2: scalability. *BMJ*. 2002;325(7372): 1090–3. https://doi.org/10.1136/bmj.325.7372.1090.

10. Benson, T. Why general practitioners use computers and hospital doctors do not – part 1: incentives. *BMJ*. 2002;325(7372): 1086–9. https://doi.org/10.1136/bmj.325.7372.1086.

11. Wachter, R. M. *Making IT Work: Harnessing the Power of Health Information: Technology to Improve Care in England*. Report of the National Advisory Group on Health Information Technology in England. Department of Health. 2016. p. 19.

12. Detmer, D., Wyatt, J., Buchan, I. National-scale clinical information exchange in the United Kingdom: lessons for the United States. *JAMIA*. 2011;18: 91–8. https://doi.org/10.1136/jamia.2010.005611.

13. Justinia, T. The UK's National Programme for IT: why was it dismantled? *Health Serv. Manage. Res.* 2016;30(1): 2–9. https://doi.org/10.1177/0951484816662492.

14. European Commission. Communication from the Commission to the European Parliament, the Council, the European Economic and Social Committee and the Committee of the Regions on enabling the

digital transformation of health and care in the digital single market; empowering citizens and building a healthier society. Brussels: European Commission. 2018. Available at: https://eur-lex.europa.eu/legal-content/EN/TXT/PDF/?uri=CELEX:52018DC0233 (accessed 16 June 2023).

15. American Psychiatric Association (APA). *Telepsychiatry via Videoconferencing: Resource Document*. Washington, DC: APA. 1998. Available at: https://citeseerx.ist.psu.edu/viewdoc/download?doi=10.1.1.173.2939&rep=rep1&type=pdf (accessed 9 January 2022).

16. American Psychiatric Association (APA). History of telepsychiatry. *Vimeo*. 17 February 2016. Available at: https://vimeo.com/155763287 (accessed 9 January 2022).

17. Blainey, G. *The Tyranny of Distance: How Distance Shaped Australia's History*. Pan Macmillan. 2010.

18. Chan, S., Parish, M., Yellowlees, P. Telepsychiatry today. *Curr. Psychiatry Rep.* 2015;17(11): 89. https://doi.org/10.1007/s11920-015-0630-9.

19. Mental Health Reform. *Rapid Briefing for the COVID-19 Crisis*. 14 April 2020. Available at: www.mentalhealthreform.ie/wp-content/uploads/2020/04/eMEN-rapid-briefing-paper_-COVID-19_final-12.pdf (accessed 9 January 2022).

20. Duerr, H. A. Making telepsychiatry work for you and your patients. *Psychiatric Times*. 22 May 2020. Available at: www.psychiatrictimes.com/view/making-telepsychiatry-work-you-and-your-patients (accessed 9 January 2022).

21. TalentLMS. The evolution and history of e-learning. n.d. Available at: www.talentlms.com/elearning/history-of-elearning (accessed 9 January 2022).

22. The Open University. The Open University. n.d. Available at: www.open.ac.uk/ (accessed 9 January 2022).

23. Coursera.n.d. Available at: www.coursera.org/ (accessed 9 January 2022).

24. Blackboard. n.d. Available at: www.blackboard.com/en-eu (accessed 9 January 2022).

25. Moodle. Moodle – open-source learning platform. n.d. Available at: https://moodle.org/ (accessed 9 January 2022).

26. Ellaway, R., Masters, K. *E-Learning in Medical Education*. Dundee: Association for Medical Education in Europe. 2008.

27. O'Shea, C., Lenihan, F, Semple, S. Abstract number: 39. Dungeons, dragons, and forensic psychiatry: improving induction for new trainees through text-based adventure games. (Conference poster). Available at: www.rcpsych.ac.uk/docs/default-source/events/competing-interests/conference-book–poster-abstracts.pdf?sfvrsn=d8734492_2 (accessed 9 January 2022).

28. Creative Commons. Marking your work with a CC license. n.d. Available at: https://wiki.creativecommons.org/wiki/Marking_your_work_with_a_CC_license (accessed 9 January 2022).

29. Full Fabric. How to design visual learning resources for neurodiverse students. n.d. Available at: www.fullfabric.com/articles/how-to-design-visual-learning-resources-for-neurodiverse-students (accessed 9 January 2022).

30. Parliamentary Office of Science and Technology (POST). *Government IT Projects*. London: POST, p. 4. 2003. Available at: www.parliament.uk/globalassets/documents/post/pr200.pdf (accessed 9 January 2022).

31. Wayner, P. The biggest software failures in recent history. *Computerworld*. 17 February 2020. Available at: www.computerworld.com/article/3412197/top-software-failures-in-recent-history.html (accessed 9 January 2022).

32. Parliamentary Office of Science and Technology. *Government IT Projects*. London: Crown, pp. 3–4. 2003. Available at: www.parliament.uk/globalassets/documents/post/pr200.pdf (accessed 9 January 2022).

33. Wachter, R. *The Digital Doctor: Hope, Hype, and Harm at the Dawn of Medicine's*

Computer Age. New York: McGraw Hill. 2015.

34. Wachter, R. M. *Making IT Work: Harnessing the Power of Health Information: Technology to Improve Care in England. Report of the National Advisory Group on Health Information Technology in England*. Department of Health. 2016.

35. Dolfing, H. Case study 1: the £10 billion IT disaster at the NHS. *Henrico Dolfing – Interim Management and Project Recovery*. 20 January 2019. Available at: www .henricodolfing.com/2019/01/case-study-1 0-billion-it-disaster.html (accessed 9 January 2022).

36. Coiera, E. W. (2007, January 1). Lessons from the NHS National Programme for IT. *Med. J. Aust.* 2007;186(1): 3–4. https://doi .org/10.5694/j.1326-5377.2007.tb00774.x.

37. Robertson, A., Bates, D. W., Sheikh, A. The rise and fall of England's National Programme for IT. *J. R. Soc. Med.* 2011;104 (11): 434–5. https://doi.org/10.1258/jrsm .2011.11k039.

38. Gould, M. NHSX moves on. Blog on the NHS Transformation Directorate website.

2022. Available at: https://transform .england.nhs.uk/blogs/nhsx-moves-on/ (accessed 6 October 2022).

39. West, E. G. Adam Smith's two views on the division of labour. *Economica* 1964;31(121): 23–32. https://doi.org/10.2307/2550924.

40. Lenihan, F. *Computers in Psychiatry*. 1st ed. London: Gaskell. 2006.

41. History of Data Science. AI winter: the highs and lows of artificial intelligence. 24 November 2021. Available at: www .historyofdatascience.com/ai-winter-the-highs-and-lows-of-artificial-intelligence/ (accessed 9 January 2022).

42. Buranyi, S. Rise of the racist robots: how AI is learning all our worst impulses. *The Guardian*, 8 August 2017. Available at: w ww.theguardian.com/inequality/2017/aug/ 08/rise-of-the-racist-robots-how-ai-is-learning-all-our-worst-impulses (accessed 9 January 2022).

43. The Royal Society. *Explainable AI: The Basics*. 2019. Available at: https://royalsoci ety.org/-/media/policy/projects/explain able-ai/AI-and-interpretability-policy-briefing.pdf (accessed 9 January 2022).

Technology-Enabled Care

Donald J Macintyre

Introduction

This chapter will focus on (1) the strategic use of technology at the public interface; (2) those considerations that will aid in determining what developments should be prioritised, and more importantly, avoided; (3) the processes and constraints which are likely to pertain when implementing developments in practice. Finally, it will explore some more, and less, successful examples.

Why Develop Technology-Enabled Mental Health Services?

Public Expectations

With the growing recognition of 'mental health', the scope of public expectations for primary care and mental health services has broadened to include not just mental illness and treatment, but also: prevention of ill health; fostering wellbeing; managing distress; supporting recovery; and building individual and community resilience. The public expects both equality of access to an adequate standard of care and that services focus on at-risk and hard-to-reach groups. The public want to be involved in decisions about their care as equal partners and for services to work closely together and share their health data when that would improve their care. They expect rapid access to safe evidence-based treatments[1] and extra support at times of transition. People with lived experience have good reason to expect to be involved in, or preferably play a leading role in, service design.

Policy Priorities

The many public priorities are reflected in government policy, embodied in mental health and suicide prevention strategies, in the findings of public inquiries into mental health services, in Covid-19 transition and recovery plans, and in commissioning guidance. Of particular note are policy aspirations to integrate local and national services, for service developments to reflect patient pathways rather than organisational boundaries and, where possible, to contain mental health activity within primary care.

In report after report, recurrent cross-cutting themes are the organisational salience of strategic (rather than reactive) service design, the crucial importance of clarity of governance, strong clinical leadership, meaningful engagement with staff and patients, recruitment and retention, workforce planning, rigorous evaluation, continuous quality improvement, use of near-real-time data, clear coordinated public communication and the fostering of organisational cultures or learning (rather than blame).

These are crucial elements for the delivery of high-quality sustainable health services, and technology-enabled care (TEC) is more likely to succeed in environments which embody these qualities and more likely to be useful if it supports them.

Evidence

Whilst the rational and humane use of data and technology in psychiatry is at least a hundred years old,[2] as can be anticipated, evidence underpinning the use of technology-enabled mental healthcare is more recent (mostly confined to the first two decades of the twenty-first century) and is expanding rapidly. However, good-quality evidence of safety and efficacy (i.e. reviews of randomised controlled trials) takes a long time to develop, so is not available for the newest technologies. In addition, digital technologies evolve at such pace that the on average seven-year delay between funding and publication of randomised controlled trials makes the results (for that specific technology) obsolete. Flexibility regarding methods of evaluation of TEC is urgently needed,[3] as is recognition of this imperative by national clinical guideline groups if their noble endeavours are to avoid being widely undermined.

Despite the methodological issues mentioned above, there is a strong mature evidence base to support remote communications technologies in mental health ('telepsychiatry').[4] Use of both telephone and videoconferencing is proven for psychiatric assessment, management and individual psychotherapy, and their widespread adoption by necessity during the pandemic has demonstrated this beyond doubt. Like all treatment options, no intervention suits everybody, and patients should have a choice if at all possible – because treatment is more successful when chosen by the patient. Whatever method is selected initially, its continued suitability should not be assumed, but kept under explicit review at every contact. In general, there is evidence of equal or better reliability, cost-effectiveness and patient and provider satisfaction compared with that found with 'in-person' therapy, particularly for common mental health problems like depression and anxiety. Evidence supports the use of telepsychiatry in hard-to-reach groups like military veterans, prisoners, some of those in ethnic minorities, and in rural areas, suggesting that videoconferencing could significantly reduce inequality by improving access. However, there are indications in some, but not all, studies that group psychotherapy is not acceptable when conducted remotely.[5]

Digital therapies underpinned by established theoretical models are safe, but more acceptable and effective when combined with human support. Online peer support is effective, but for safety requires human moderation. Mobile, smartphone-enabled care, with or without passive sensing, may eventually become ubiquitous, but today this evidence base is still developing.[6] Whilst therapeutic gaming is in its infancy, virtual reality has demonstrated real promise in those with low literacy and in treating anxiety and phobia. Clinical evidence supporting the use of avatar therapy in psychosis is developing. Scripted chatbots (and those claiming to use artificial intelligence) have great potential, but at the time of writing are lacking in robust clinical evidence; some have overpromised and underdelivered, been used in populations for which they have not been developed or had significant doubts raised over their safety.[7]

An indication of the applicability of evidence-based TEC in mental health settings is summarised in Figure 2.1.

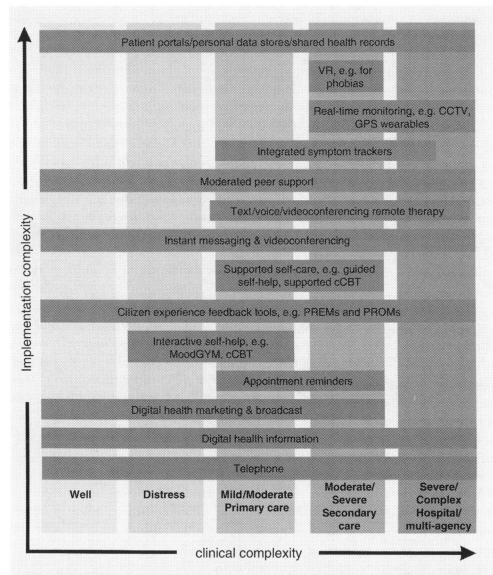

Figure 2.1 Safe and effective mental health technology-enabled care

Undoubtedly, new technologies will be adopted by some in a haphazard manner, and their use expanded outside their proper indications, causing waste and harm. If we are to avoid contributing to the chaos, we must balance enthusiasm and flexibility with caution and scepticism.

Resources

Excluding the pandemic, the last 10 years have seen a real-term stagnation in health spending in the UK, and it seems likely that the financial situation will not change radically for the better in the foreseeable future. Furthermore, there is a worldwide shortage of clinical personnel, and high rates of burnout, long-term sickness absence and early retirement in these professional groups. That means we must do more with about the same financial resources as we have at present (i.e. increase productivity) by making the best use of the time of our existing clinicians, by being flexible about expanding the roles of staff without clinical registration and by making concerted and sustained efforts to allow those with a wealth of lived experience to participate in supporting their peers and building their own resilience and that of their communities. Blending this increasing diversity of human resource with the right technology, where that reduces waste and improves quality, has the potential to be the force multiplier we need.

Several caveats are worth mentioning: firstly, we should be modest about what health services can achieve alone – long-term cohort studies (of, for example, British civil servants and residents of Framingham, Massachusetts and Almeda County, California) have estimated that only about 10 per cent of overall health is determined by health services, compared with genetics (30%), environmental conditions (5%) and social determinants such as education and inequality (15%). Having said that, in these studies, the remaining and largest category of determinants of health was 'behavioural' (40%) – this category represents 'the daily choices we make with respect to diet, physical activity, and sex; the substance abuse and addictions to which we fall prey; our approach to safety; and our coping strategies in confronting stress',[8] and may therefore in theory be influenced by health and care services.

Secondly, the adoption of technology in healthcare, rather than decreasing the overall cost of care, tends to increase it – so all proposed TEC developments should be carefully costed and considered within the overall budget of providing care for a given population. If the overall budget is to remain fairly fixed, to secure resources for new developments less productive (lower-quality) activities will need to cease; the fate of sacred cows may need reconsidering, and difficult decisions cannot be avoided – a 'value-based healthcare' framework may help structure these discussions.[9]

Which Initiatives Should We Prioritise When Considering Technology-Enabled Mental Healthcare?

There are endless possible ways in which services can be improved, and those wishing to lead change must contend with the many well-meaning but naive suggestions to buy or build an app, set up a helpline or launch a new website or an 'awareness-raising' social media campaign. These crosswinds can be resisted by setting out a clear well-justified alternative vision, built on a broad overview of population-level unmet need, viewing current services and proposed developments from citizens' (or 'the user') perspective, and mapping common patient or user journeys from health, through distress and illness, to recovery.

Need

It is likely to be difficult to establish what the level of unmet need is within a population; however, this information is foundational to building a case for change. The first step is defining the population of interest. The temptation may be to consider those likely to come into contact with a service; however, it is more meaningful to initially consider all those (i.e. 'the population') in an area or region within a diagnostic group (e.g. mood disorders) or problem group (e.g. users of unscheduled care), and determine what information is available locally and how this agrees with the published literature. This should allow a quantitative estimate of unmet need. If we are fortunate, we may be able to map individual patient journeys of those currently in contact with services, which can add hard quantitative detail. However, this information can be dry for non-specialists and can only take us so far – hard data, seasoned by representative (suitably anonymised) anecdotes, tend to be much more persuasive.

Once an estimate of unmet need has been established, it is worthwhile to consider the structure of support for our population of interest across the full spectrum of need, from friends and supporting family members, those who may be healthy but at increased risk, those in distress but not yet breaching the threshold for a clinical diagnosis, to those with mild, moderate and severe difficulties. This so-called 'stepped-care' model will be familiar to most readers and remains a useful structure in which we can place existing services, consider the quality of our evidence of unmet needs, match existing technologies and locate emerging ones. This can be a profound activity when reviewed on a regular basis, providing a firm bulwark against kneejerk initiatives which can be easily located within the model, allowing their merits to be rapidly assessed and considered within a broader strategic plan.

Another important contextual element to consider when formulating initiatives is the current sociotechnical environment.

Health Information Infrastructure/Installed Base

The existing e-health ecosystem is sometimes called the health information infrastructure (HII), and the people and platforms currently working in a health system the 'installed base'. The systems we use to deliver healthcare are an amalgamation of multiple systems of different ages and original purposes, joined together or embedded within each other, with varying degrees of success. For that reason, our workflows are often tortuous, and risky workarounds like cutting and pasting text multiple times from one application to another, or feathering our workstations with Post-it® note instructions and logins, are all too common. New developments can easily be lost in this cluttered and chaotic environment, and this is true in the public-facing domestic environment of TEC – people already have their own preferred devices, apps, habits and workflows – and any project that ignores this is destined to fail. We must acknowledge the current situation and realistically lay out how people will transition to the envisioned future. We should consider not just citizens' technical and social readiness for any initiative, but also their widely varied personal perspectives, health literacy, and the prevalence and uncertain course and outcomes of mental ill health.

Citizens' Perspectives

It may be helpful to bear in mind several fundamental facts about mental illness and care: (1) mental illness is common,* but strange to the uninitiated (*which is most*

---

* The (UK) Adult Psychiatric Morbidity Survey consistently estimates around one in six adults have a common mental disorder in any given week. https://digital.nhs.uk/data-and-information/publica tions/statistical/adult-psychiatric-morbidity-survey/adult-psychiatric-morbidity-survey-survey-of- mental-health-and-wellbeing-england-2014.

people); (2) the majority of people who experience a common mental health problem like mixed depression and anxiety *do not seek or receive any help* for the experience;[†] (3) about 90% of those who do seek help receive that assistance in primary care or non-health settings; (4) about half of those affected will *have only one episode* during their lifetime; but (5) for those who do have the misfortune to develop a recurrence of depression or anxiety, or a severe mental illness, *multiple episode are likely, and a chronic course is not uncommon.*

It can be instructive to consider how we might react if we had a panic attack for the first time, or to think about what it might be like to be asked repeatedly to explain ourselves to the (however kind) professional doing their jobs: perhaps the police, then the ambulance staff, the triage nurse, the casualty doctor and then the psychiatrist in a noisy emergency department. However empathetic we are, our personal perspective is by definition idiosyncratic; people who work in services are particularly likely to develop blind spots about them, and there are always 'unknown unknowns' – it is for these reasons that it is necessary to seek people's perspectives directly.

People who have personal experience of mental illness, and their friends and families, tend to relate their personal narratives in three main phases:

I. The first phase may be conceived of as 'finding support' – this is the stage at which symptoms, distress and impairment are occurring but the person does not understand what is wrong, does not know where to look for help and does not know what their options might be or how to choose between them. This phase is often accompanied by disabling fear and feelings of isolation and alienation, and can be prolonged.

II. Assuming the person is able to find support, at the second stage – 'experiencing support' – there may be a protracted wait for access, repeated assessments, coming to terms with the stigma and implications of a new diagnosis, mixed experiences of the support offered, new side effects of treatment, stabilisation, improvement, a growing understanding of the illness and the development of expertise in self-management.

III. The third stage – 'recovery/thriving' – encompasses recognition of what works for them, determining what ambitions to let go of, what roles or relationships to sacrifice to prioritise the hard work needed to stay well, growing confidence, perhaps a sense of mastery over their condition, the work of defining a new self-identity and renewing of responsibilities, and for many, the desire to help others who are going through something similar.

This is obviously a simplification of what is not a linear process, and those with recurrent difficulties will move back and forth between phases repeatedly – sometimes facing the same barriers to accessing support as they did the first time. We should also recognise that in more complex cases the burden of treatment is considerable, and that comorbidities, multiple supports and agencies do not add, but multiply the complexity for the patient and their family – particularly when our systems rely on the patient to communicate between agencies and coordinate scheduling!

We tend to evaluate our services using the data we have available – usually quantitative data that is collected automatically – process information which is several steps removed from what matters to individuals. But we do have one reliable source of rich qualitative

---

[†] According to the Adult Psychiatric Morbidity Survey (2014), around one in three people in the UK with common mental disorders receive treatment.

data – in the form of complaints! Nobody likes being criticised, but we know that when it comes to improving systems, critical feedback is often more helpful than praise. Even grossly unreasonable criticism tends to have a few nuggets of fair comment embedded in it, and an unflinching thematic review of complaints is likely to identify important areas for improvement. When appropriately anonymised and amalgamated, these individual user journeys can be used as strong arguments for service change.

In summary, we should consider approaches which encompass the needs of people and their supporters in each of the three phases of their 'journey' – that is (1) finding support, (2) experiencing support and (3) recovery. We should take account of and facilitate movement between phases and be mindful that the needs of those going through this for the first time will be quite different from those with recurrent difficulties. Importantly, we should recognise the enormous wealth of experience and goodwill of those in recovery and consider it an obligation to realise their desire to help others going through something similar.

Design

Design is not just about creating solutions. Using a design approach, and working with designers if you can, helps in the selection of areas for development. The Design Council's 'Double Diamond' framework, launched in 2004,[10] helpfully breaks down the design process into four phases, starting with 'Discovery' – in which need is explored in depth and with users; this allows a clarity of focus in which need is more clearly 'Defined' (the second stage); the third stage is an exploratory 'Development' of solutions, which allows a focus on a chosen solution in the final 'Delivery' phase. In practice, discovery and definition may need to be repeated, and the development and delivery phases are iterative. The model is particularly useful in resisting the precipitous rush to 'solutionising' without adequate exploration of the key issue of user need and can help oppose pressure to bring in an unsuitable but immediately available 'quick fix'.

'Empathic design' principles recognise the crucial importance of the care we must take when using technology, in order to foster and preserve trust, consider the dignity and feelings of our patients and maintain high ethical standards (e.g. regarding the secondary use of data).

Designers are experts at user engagement, and they find creative ways to involve people, not just in thinking about a particular technology, but in exploring the whole patient journey. They will jump at the chance to work with the public on something that matters, synthesising the user perspective and presenting it visually, with the kind of immediate impact that cannot be made in writing.

There should be no excuse to avoid including users in design discussions from the outset, and as the design develops their meaningful involvement increases the likelihood of securing funding, improves external legitimacy, reduces the risk of a major failure, improves experiences of care and results in better clinical outcomes.

Process Mapping

Rather than designing a service from scratch, we are often faced with redesigning services; quality improvement models that have industrial legacies (e.g. Lean, Six Sigma, Toyota) can conceptualise healthcare as a form of 'production' – a model which could be appropriate for procedures such as endoscopy, elective surgery or electro-convulsive therapy (ECT). These industrial models are less relevant when applied to unscheduled and drawn-out recursive health and care processes, which depend to a great extent on the active participation of the patient and their family. Nevertheless, process mapping can be a useful part of the discovery phase of any redesign,[11] as no individual has knowledge of every step of a patient pathway. Process mapping has many potential benefits – it tends to uncover hidden complexities, reveal under-appreciated redundancies, foster understanding across departmental and institutional boundaries, and promote a shared lexicon.

User Archetypes and Universal Barriers to Access

Imagined stereotypical users (known as archetypes or personae) are used in design to represent common or challenging presentations. Thinking about how archetypes might interact with a pathway (particularly when those stereotypes are based on real-world data) can improve anticipation of the varying needs of a diverse population, reducing the risk that false assumptions contribute to failure or inequity. When redesigning services to integrate technology-enabled elements, we should consider the pathway for non-English speakers, those with sensory or cognitive impairments, or those with physical disabilities. We are all likely to have to live with functional impairments through some part of our lives – designs which are suitable for people with a range of abilities tend to improve accessibility for everybody: for example, the dropped kerbs mandated by disability legislation make life easier for elderly people, parents with young children and those recovering from traumatic injuries.

When considering access to TEC, data-driven archetypes or real-life user stories can be particularly powerful when viewed in conjunction with cross-cutting themes that designers have identified by analysing many user stories.[12] These so-called 'universal barriers to access' (Table 2.1) increase the burden of treatment or inhibit the individual from initiating action; minimising these barriers should be an important goal during the development phase.

Summary

Using data and public engagement can enable us to establish clearly the need for change. Use of archetypes and real users' stories helps us define our goals and priorities. Working with users and designers can help mitigate major risks, establish clear aims and focus, set a clear direction of travel and build a firm foundation for change which will stand up to external scrutiny. Now we move from 'what?' to 'how?'

Table 2.1 Universal barriers to access

UNIVERSAL BARRIERS TO ACCESS
1. time – e.g. waiting, travelling, form filling
2. finance – e.g. lost earnings, travel expenses, data charges
3. (physical) access – e.g. to an office, a printer, a scanner
4. interface/interaction capability – e.g. reading and writing ability, computer skills
5. self-confidence – e.g. to fill in a long form, cope with uncertainty
6. awareness – e.g. that a service exists, of the opening hours, the phone number
7. comprehension – e.g. to retain information, to navigate signage
8. emotional state – e.g. to have the drive and resilience to take on a new task
9. trust – e.g. in authority figures, in security of disclosure of sensitive information
10. (physical) evidence – e.g. bank statements, doctors' letters, identification
11. enthusiasm – e.g. to try something online, to ask for help

How Do We Increase the Likelihood of Successfully Implementing Technology-Enabled Care Projects?

As our politicians demonstrate, success can be defined in many ways. Most of us on reflection will probably conclude that success is about creating sustainable positive change. Although we may be prepared to dedicate a significant proportion of our lives to a project, the will to succeed is necessary but not sufficient, and there are many potential pitfalls to be avoided. This section focuses on likely and potential hurdles to successful sustained development.

Complexity and Failure

Literature has been emerging over the last decade which considers failures of broad technological and organisational change. One approach, termed the 'NASSS framework', examines non-adoption (N), abandonment (A), scale-up (S), spread (S) and sustainability (S) issues. This framework is a useful way to consider TEC projects – across seven domains, in each of which the complexity of a development can be graded at one of three levels: as 'simple (straightforward, predictable, few components), complicated (multiple interacting components or issues), or complex (dynamic, unpredictable, not easily disaggregated into constituent components). Programs characterized by complicatedness proved difficult but not impossible to implement' (p 392). Projects displaying 'complexity in multiple NASSS domains rarely, if ever' (p. 401),[13] succeeded.[‡] There are many lessons to learn here, including that success is less about technology and much more about people and culture; and that careful strategic thinking, good leadership, wide stakeholder engagement and the identification and mitigation of risk are essential.

Strategy and Leadership

Talking about strategy and leadership can feel awkward and pretentious, and there are many bad business books that are like this. Nevertheless, strategy and leadership do matter and must be addressed in any proposal. 'Strategic plans' often confuse aims and objectives, and targets and lists of ongoing projects, with 'strategy'. Strategic thinking is about (1) clearly defining the nature of the challenge – taking a complex situation and identifying which are the critical aspects which require focus; (2) clearly articulating the main principles which will guide responses to the challenge;[§] and (3) developing a set of coherent actions – which are *coordinated and mutually reinforcing* (and need careful planning to implement). It will be evident that delivering a strategy requires leadership (to communicate a clear vision, make critical decisions and hold the authority to allocate the necessary resources), clarity of roles and responsibilities, broad engagement and cooperation with key stakeholders, and coordination of activity, often across teams, departments and organisations. A good place to start is with stakeholders.

Stakeholders

This term refers to all those who need to be consulted for the project to succeed; they will change over time. Whilst the public should be consulted throughout, and at the risk of stating the obvious, it is crucial to identify early on those people who can permit or, more

---

[‡] Creating a vaccine is complicated; suicide prevention is complex.
[§] One cannot afford to have too many main principles as they will quickly conflict. An important personal principle is to play to your strengths – build your team to compensate for your weaknesses.

importantly, block a project and bring them on side. These 'key stakeholders' are, for example, chief executives, heads of IT departments, information governors, chairs of Royal Colleges or other important committees, and sometimes senior civil servants and politicians – all ambitious, busy people with many competing responsibilities, priorities and agendas. What they share is a desire to improve the lives of the public, deliver successful projects and receive credit for doing so. It is vital to develop and publicly rehearse an 'elevator pitch' which you can deploy whenever you get the opportunity of a few minutes of their valuable time. Think about how this pitch can be framed so that you can emphasise how this project helps them nobly meet their goals and priorities – to do this, you need to find out what these are![14] Focus your efforts on those who may be sceptical, but whose support is critical – you do not need to preach to the converted. It is better to start at the top of organisational hierarchies and work down than try to work up. If you can, include stakeholders as co-authors on proposals and state clearly how they will contribute to the success of the project. Be generous (but honest and sincere) in praising your stakeholders – acknowledge their support and their specific contribution publicly, and include them, for example, as co-presenters at important meetings. When you have developed a successful pitch and a network of stakeholders, it is time to write a business case.

Business Case Development

A 'business case' (case = justification) can take many forms. Ultimately it is a document designed to justify the risk and expense of your project. Full business cases are long, highly detailed documents, whilst outline (strategic) business cases can be two-page summaries. Like grant applications, there are three main domains which are essential to address to satisfy critical readers: (1) the merits of the project itself, including the degree of alignment between the project's ambitions and the resources (including time) requested to deliver it; (2) the suitability of the skills and experience, commitment and availability of the project team; and (3) the strength and engagement of the institutional support structures in which the team and project will be embedded. Writing a business case will be easier if you follow a logical sequence:

- Start with why change is needed.
- Set the strategic context and describe how this project is aligned.
- Describe your user engagement and how this sits within your stakeholder network.
- Present your vision and goals – this could include alternatives ranging from modest to radical change.
- Describe how things will change – the transformation your project will make to the user experience, to processes and systems.
- Describe the structures and assets the project will use to deliver the change, for example, workforce, estates and technology.
- Explain the operating or logic model of delivery, with attention to who, what, when, where, why and how. Will you use an Agile/iterative method?
- Lay out a delivery sequence, with a timeline, description of a minimum viable product and the fully realised system; include public communication and project evaluation.

For detailed (cf. outline) business cases, create an executive summary – this is the most important section, as most people will never read the whole document. Aim for a narrative structure, concision and clarity. A good executive summary should give the reader a clear impression of the project's complexity because, as we saw earlier, complexity is associated with failure. Do not be tempted to gloss over any flaws – there are always risks, but these can be mitigated. If there are several, do you need a rethink?

Assuming your business case clears its last hurdle and is finally given the green light, you can expect your celebrations to be short-lived as you suddenly feel the weight of responsibility to publicly deliver on your ambitions! You are going to need help – a lot of it – and programme and project management will be an essential element.

Programme and Project Management

In the hierarchy of change management, projects are distinct activities consisting of many related changes; programmes are bundles of projects, and portfolios are made of several programmes. Programme (also known as service development) managers and project managers are the unsung heroes of successful development.

Like any profession, they have their own culture and argot; they use arcane methods like 'MSP', 'PRINCE2', 'Scrum' and 'Kanban' – structured processes (models of implementation) with their own accreditation schemes, prophets, manifestos, disciples and heretics. The main schism is between more modern so-called 'Agile' and traditional 'waterfall' methods. Waterfall models of project management tend to operate over long cycles (years), with highly detailed specifications and unwieldy tendering processes, delivering stodgy off-the-peg enterprise systems from multinational brand name suppliers. By contrast, Agile methodologies, beloved of our social media overlords, 'move fast and break things':[**] these are software development techniques, operating over much shorter cycles, highly focused on user need and engagement, with rapidly evolving products that are never truly complete.[15] The larger the project, the more focused on procurement, infrastructure and on enterprise (office desktop) applications, the more likely it is to use waterfall methods. Conversely, for public-facing TEC projects, it is likely that Agile methods will play a part, particularly when it comes to the software development phase. High levels of agility are difficult to achieve in healthcare settings because serious clinical and information governance risks require a measured approach.

In either case, good programme and project management is vital to the success of digital development and implementation. Project managers create and sustain the infrastructure that brings together the user researchers, designers, developers, clinicians, finance, operation managers, communication, marketing, risk management, action logs, meetings and schedules and the documents which help a project succeed, and neglecting to include them in a business case or budget is a schoolboy error. Another regrettably frequent but grave error is to fail to give adequate priority to matters of cybersecurity and information governance.

Information Governance and Cybersecurity

Information governance issues are amongst the most vexing and time-consuming potential obstacles and should be standing items on a project agenda, attended to as early as possible. A working knowledge of the GDPR (General Data Protection Regulation) principles is a significant advantage, and extra scrutiny should be given to issues of 'special category data' (e.g. concerning health) and the lawful bases for processing, particularly consent, because 'Public authorities . . . may find it more difficult to show valid freely given consent.'[16]

[**] Internal motto used by Facebook until 2014.

Caldicott guardians and information governance officers cannot be co-applicants on a project, but they are key stakeholders, particularly at the start of the project, and should be cultivated, shown respect and given plenty of time to make decisions. They are in an invidious position, for they receive no praise for preventing disasters, only blame for permitting them, and they have little incentive to make a quick decision or err on the side of taking risks. They have a high degree of autonomy, and their rulings can sometimes appear arbitrary. Filling in Data Protection Impact Assessment (DPIA) forms in fine detail takes precious time, but not as much as appealing an unfavourable decision. Time invested early in informal discussions seeking guidance on 'how do we make this work?' is infinitely more effective than submitting a late application with a covering note stating 'this is our grand plan – please would you approve it ASAP?'

The scope of DPIAs should be carefully framed: neither over-encompassing (data collection must be justified on the grounds of improving patient outcomes and experience) nor excessively narrow. For example, it is important to share patient data where it would improve patient care, and services justifiably need to be able to share personal identifiers across institutional boundaries, such as for public protection, to support those with complex psychosocial needs and to continuously improve the quality of the patient journey.

Whilst information governance issues are particularly crucial in the initial stages, security issues gradually grow in importance and continue after the project has left the development phase.

As ransomware attacks on critical health infrastructure have shown, cybersecurity is, or should be, a concern for our whole society. We have all been entreated to keep our devices updated, to use secure passwords, enable two-factor authentication, and be sceptical about embedded links, attachments and offers that sound too good to be true. Security and usability are often in tension; however, designing with users can mitigate security risks such as insecure workarounds – like reusing passwords – by taking human factors into consideration. For example, allowing longer passwords which change infrequently reduces the cognitive load required to frequently generate and remember new passwords, reduces password reuse and results in passwords that are much harder to crack.

Online fraud and extortion continue to be low-risk and high-reward pursuits, conducted with impunity, often from within rogue states; the problem is growing rapidly with no end in sight. For TEC, this raises issues of trust, uptake, reputation and clinical risk management in both the development and deployment of health IT systems.

Clinical Risk Management

Clinical risk management standards and processes are less stodgy and more practical than they sound – they provide assurance that technology-enabled changes will be safe, and build and maintain public trust. This is a rapidly evolving area, and there is debate about whether international (ISO) or national standards should be used. In England, there are two main sets of standards which cover the manufacture (DCB0129) and deployment (DCB0160) of health and care IT systems which could potentially cause harm to patients, including those classified as a medical device (see the following section). They do not cover cybersecurity or information governance. These standards are mandatory in England, and are regarded as good practice in the rest of the UK.

Central to the standards is the role of the Clinical Safety Officer (CSO), who must be a suitably qualified and experienced clinician and who is responsible for ensuring that the standards are followed. CSO training can be completed over a day or two,[17] provides a framework for risk analysis and management and can significantly reduce the risk of design flaws or user error causing catastrophic failure. The frameworks also provide a structure to document and justify decisions – which could prove very useful should the worst happen.

The two main phases of clinical risk management are (I) proactive anticipation and mitigation and (II) effective monitoring and resolution of emerging risks. The first phase requires (a) identification of potential but realistic hazards, (b) evaluating the risk (hazard severity × likelihood) and then (c) determining what mitigation is required (risk control).

Importantly, it is envisaged that the CSO is not expected to conduct these procedures independently, but is responsible for facilitating the project team to think through these processes together in a workshop setting, with the focus being on what could go wrong at each stage of the patient journey,[††] and capturing these and their mitigations in a 'Hazard Log'. Evaluating risk is a matter of judgement and humans can be very bad at making these judgements, as the gambling and finance industries can attest. It is important to take a measured and balanced approach to prevent a highly risk-averse minority from having undue influence.

The 'Clinical Safety Case Report' presents the arguments and supporting evidence that provides a justification that a system is safe at that time and should be available for the 'Go-Live' decision and updated as the project progresses. A suggested report structure makes it clear that this is not to be undertaken lightly,[18] but it is hard to argue that either the standards, processes or their components are unnecessary.

The scope of clinical risk management standards includes medical devices, which have their own additional regulatory framework.

Medical Devices

In technology-enabled mental healthcare, most 'devices' are not physical products, but rather software or apps. The legislation governing these devices is evolving, but at the time of writing the Medicines and Healthcare products Regulatory Agency (MHRA) plays a lead role. If you are developing software that has a 'medical purpose', such as a diagnostic or therapeutic role, it might fall under medical device regulation – however, this is a grey area and depends to some extent on the exact use of language.[19] This is important for our purposes, as psychological approaches may not be considered 'medical'. Health and wellbeing devices are unlikely to be included, and the regulations may not apply to a device only being used within the institute it was made but if you are intending to give the device to another institution, or any commercial marketing is planned, it is likely the regulations will apply and UK Conformity Assessed marking (which replaces CE marking in the UK) will be needed.

If you are not developing a custom solution, but rather are procuring an existing product, you will need to evaluate the options.

Evaluating Technology

We have already touched on off-the-peg technological solutions and noted that these are often marketed strongly and can become hazardous if they attract naive but influential champions; however, if you have identified a clear need and taken into account the detailed wider context, you may determine that such a solution is warranted. In that case, you will

---

[††] Again we see the crucial importance of process mapping and user archetypes.

need to evaluate the options using a structured approach, working with your stakeholders and the procurement team.

The exact process will vary but at some stage you will be part of a group scoring suppliers' submissions, which are likely to include evidence from the supplier about their service in fine detail across multiple domains. One approach,[20] intended to simplify this process, includes sections on company information, the value proposition,[‡‡] clinical safety, data protection, technical security, interoperability, usability and accessibility. However, it is wise to also consider more widely how the technology will be implemented – like any business case or a grant application, one needs to consider not just the intervention, but also the institutional context and the capacity of the team available.[§§] A strong supplier submission will should include evidence of:

1. *Effectiveness*, the similarities and differences between your population and those previously studied, and how evidence of effectiveness will be continuously demonstrated during the life of the project.
2. *Feasibility*, including (a) evidence of successful implementation, preferably in a context as close to your own as possible; the extent to which in these other contexts the core components of service have been identified and defined, in terms of service model, technical requirements, implementation strategy, ongoing clinical governance, information governance, clinical buy-in, evaluation protocol and communication/ marketing strategy; (b) product usage data, dropout and completion rates, recorded complaints and adverse events.
3. *Support*, which includes (a) product support (offered by the supplier directly to users), evidence that this will be provided in a timely manner, and a commitment that the supplier will continue to cooperate to develop, evaluate and improve the product; (b) service support during implementation, including technical support and logistical advice and documentary support; (c) training that will be available during implementation and operation.
4. *Need*, in your population, that this need will be met in the target population, that the product meets service or system gaps, and clarity that this will either be an add-on or a replacement.
5. *Fit*, (a) of the service, in terms of alignment with national strategic priorities and delivery in a stepped/matched care model or in a multidisciplinary team approach; evidence of clinical and technical support from within key stakeholder groups, together with ease of integration into existing governance and reporting structures; (b) technical fit, in terms of interoperability with existing patient management systems.
6. *Site capacity*, which includes financial, staff, administrative, technical, training and information governance capacity.

Evaluating technology options takes time, is a group activity and requires senior clinical, operational and technical input. If you are fortunate to have a range of supplier bids, using this type of framework will allow you to score each bid, use a weighting system for each category to calculate the overall score, rank the options and select a winner for procurement, local implementation and, in concert, marketing and communication.

---

‡‡ Why a user should purchase a good or service, and how that that value will be delivered.
§§ These criteria were developed by Chris Wright, National Advisor for Digital Mental Health, Scottish Government, and are based on the National Implementation Research Network (NIRN) Hexagon Tool.

Marketing and Communication

Marketing and communication are closely related, and the terms are often used interchangeably. The term 'marketing' implies the goal is not just to inform, but to also influence behaviour, and has more commercial overtones. Marketing could be defined as the strategic use of communication. Good marketing and communications can have a dramatic impact on reputation and access, and they are vital elements of TEC projects. On the contrary, poor planning and marketing implementation can have an equally deleterious effect. The most important risk is that a mismatch will develop between a project's capacity and demand, and that as a result the project cannot deliver on its promises. This may occur as demand rises when premature news of a project begins to diffuse organically, for example, as a result of an over-enthusiastic funder or senior sponsor. Alternatively, supply may be compromised, for example, by dependence at a vital step on a single individual who becomes unexpectedly unavailable. A marketing strategy is a core part of implementation, and careful choreography is required to balance supply and demand.

For TEC projects, it is likely that much of the marketing will be done digitally. Most organisations have communication teams, which have more or less in-house digital marketing expertise, and may have strong links or existing contracts with commercial advertising agencies. It may be best to build on this arrangement. On the one hand, advertising agencies have large contracts with social media companies, and if there is a problem with a campaign (for example, an account is locked out or an advert is mistakenly classified by AI as inappropriate), it is likely the agency can pick up the phone and speak to someone in the social media company to quickly resolve an issue, whereas an in-house campaign is unlikely to have that kind of technical support. However, despite the lower quality of technical support, and the potential conflict it could cause between a project and its comms colleagues, there are a number of good reasons why it may be advantageous to bring digital marketing in house on TEC projects: firstly, direct control of any communications is significantly more agile than working through a relationship with a third party controlled by another team; secondly, digital teams may have some members already with significant experience in digital marketing; thirdly (if internal resources can be continually dedicated), an in-house campaign is likely to be an order of magnitude more cost-effective than using an agency; finally, an in-house campaign has immediate access to all the data generated by the campaign, which is vital for quality improvement, particularly when combined with user research and testing – and again, this is best done within the project team.

An envious quantity of interesting data is generated by a digital marketing campaign, and its immediacy is startling – a live digital dashboard allows iterative approaches to be quickly tested and refined. This data should form part of the evaluation of any project, and it can be used for quality improvement and research.

Service Evaluation, Quality Improvement and Research

Service evaluation, audit, quality improvement and research are easy bedfellows, as they require similar skills, methods and mindsets. Although their boundaries can blur, their purposes are fairly distinct, and it is necessary to distinguish research from audit and service evaluation for reasons of ethical governance.[21] Research 'attempts to derive generalisable or transferable new knowledge', whereas service evaluation is 'conducted solely to define or judge current care' and audit 'measures against a [predetermined] standard'.[22] Collecting and analysing data for service development and quality improvement activity (designed with the intention of directly improving patient care) is likely to be considered service evaluation. Whilst this is very unlikely to require formal research ethical approval, some local scrutiny may be necessary depending on the setting, and as mentioned previously, it is prudent to discuss a project's data retention and analysis plans with information governance colleagues to avoid the unwelcome prospect of unexpected DPIAs.

Some thought to evaluation is needed at the inception of a project: an evaluation plan should be mentioned in the project outline and be fleshed out in some detail in the funding application or business case.

A robust approach which is both useful and should silence reflexive naysayers and reassure nervous stakeholders is a logic model (often displayed graphically as a 'driver diagram'). Driver diagrams are structured charts of three or more levels that explain the project team's theory of how a project will achieve its goals.[23] They break down a goal into components necessary for success and individual actions, and in this way make explicit what should be included in an evaluation.

A valid, rich and persuasive evaluation should include organisational and user perspectives, using both quantitative and qualitative data to address quality measures in the six quality domains of safety: effectiveness, efficiency, timeliness, person-centredness, equality and diversity. Think about the evaluation in terms of its impacts on the organisation, as well as its intended effects. The equality and diversity impacts of a project are amongst the most challenging to evaluate as data about protected characteristics is highly sensitive (and therefore places a grave responsibility on the data processor to ensure the safety of the data), is very unlikely to be already available and, despite their importance, asking about protected characteristics may be considered an imposition by some people.

Whilst it is likely that a project will generate large quantities of process data, the majority of this will be of limited value. Consider each set of variables that will be available and whether they can tell a story in each of the quality domains – what is the most valid way of doing this? It is unhelpful to report many measures in one domain – pick the best one or two quantitative measures and include qualitative measures. If you don't already have this information in a quality domain (as is likely), you will need to collect additional data specifically for that purpose. Plan this early on – it will become incrementally harder to achieve this as the project progresses.

Creating a valid and informative evaluation will significantly increase the likelihood that a project will be judged a success and graduate to become part of 'business as usual'. If it does, good-quality metrics embedded in the design facilitate continuous quality improvement and, ultimately, sustainability.

Most projects succeed in some areas and fail in others. Examining case studies can be instructive.

Technology-Enabled Care Case Studies

Dementia Post-Diagnostic Support Platform

Adapting to a new diagnosis of dementia is often distressing and brings with it many uncertainties for the patient and their family. Policy aspiration was that everyone with a new diagnosis of dementia should be offered up to a year of post-diagnostic support from mental health services or third sector organisations, but capacity to provide this fell short by about 50%. A proposal was developed to provide a technology-enabled support platform that bundled together three packages for people with a recent diagnosis of dementia and their families. The platform was comprised of an online dementia information hub, a carer and family support app and a home care management package, either installed on existing devices or provided on a free tablet with data bundle. Use of the platform by people living with dementia and their families was lower than anticipated. An analysis of the project identified that many individuals with dementia either did not identify with the diagnosis or became frustrated or distressed when the diagnosis was raised. Others were already moderately demented at diagnosis, thus limiting the value of some components. Some families thought elements of the platform could be valuable, but not at that time. In dementia, early introduction of technology may be important even when the intervention may not be *effective* until a change in circumstances occurs. Longitudinal engagement with families is likely to be necessary to achieve the potential benefits of TEC.[24]

In retrospect, two fundamental and related weaknesses were likely to have been responsible for the failure of the intervention: (1) a technology and provider centric perspective had been taken during the design process and (2) the preferences and needs of service users hadn't been adequately taken into account. Time pressure to design and deliver an intervention as quickly as possible also contributed to the failure to place people living with dementia and their families at the centre of the design process. Excessive complexity of the intervention was a likely contributory factor, as was a lack of personalisation.

To address these issues, TEC for people living with dementia and their families should (1) have been considered as part of a wider redesign of post-diagnostic support, (2) should have been co-designed with service users and other relevant stakeholders and (3) should have focused on personalising care and support.

Webchat Introduction in a Telephone-Centric Service

A mental wellbeing crisis listening service decided to explore adding a webchat channel to its telephone-based service. It introduced the technology in a 'soft launch', adding the service without fanfare to its website. Evaluation was conducted over several months through a series of staff interviews, pre- and post-webchat surveys, and using process data generated by the technology. It was found that 40% of demand came from outside the region, with a higher preponderance of men using webchat compared to the telephone service. Webchat users were likely to be new to the service and said they would not have phoned had webchat been unavailable. Webchat users reported a higher burden of distress and suicidality. Although webchat took two to three times longer than telephone interactions, it was decided to continue the webchat service for an additional year, during which time the Covid-19 pandemic emerged. During the pandemic, resource restrictions increased, and provision of telephone services were prioritised.

Here, a new technology was introduced in an informal manner without a clear value proposition; the evaluation demonstrated an acute user need but not cost-effectiveness. The organisational context of the new service was one of limited resilience. It is difficult to sustain projects with high complexity in multiple domains. An evaluation which does not fully address the main quality indicators reduces the likelihood of sustainable development.

Digital Marketing of Web-based Services

Unlimited licences were procured for digital mental wellbeing interactive courses and made available to mental health services. A patient information website conducted user research which indicated people were uncertain about the meaning of 'wellbeing' and anxious about signing up for services. It created a signposting tool, designed for mobile devices, and a web page explaining the tools, what was involved in signing up and a short interactive guide to help choose between them. The website team initiated a digital marketing campaign which cost pennies to bring each person to the signposting tool. Sign-up for the interactive courses increased more than tenfold and was sustained during the campaign. Overall, the cost per user went down significantly. The cost-effectiveness of an intervention can be increased by user research and marketing.

Summary

Having ideas is easy, but implementing them is hard. The chances of success can be improved by building a broad coalition of essential stakeholders, persuading the sceptical, respecting your information governance (IG) colleagues, careful planning, and thinking about and minimising risks. Leadership, strategic thinking, persuasion, attention to detail and a team approach are needed. Professional project management, good marketing and communication are vital for implementation, and a robust evaluation is essential for sustainability.

Acknowledgements

I would like to thank Dr Ania Zubala and Chris Wright for their helpful feedback on this chapter.

References

1. Scottish Government. *Mental Health in Scotland – a 10-Year Vision: Analysis of Responses to the Public Engagement Exercise.* 2016. Available at: www.gov.scot/publications/mental-health-scotland-10-year-vision-analysis-responses-public-engagement/documents/ (accessed 20 June 2023).

2. Kraepelin, E. *Manic-Depressive Insanity and Paranoia.* Edinburgh: Livingstone. 1921.

3. Bickman, L. Improving mental health services: a 50-year journey from randomized experiments to artificial intelligence and precision mental health. *Adm. Policy Ment. Health Ment. Health Serv. Res.* 2020;47: 795–843.

4. Aboujaoude, E., Salame, W., Naim, L. Telemental health: a status update. *World Psychiatry* 2015;14: 223–30.

5. Jenkins-Guarnieri, M. A., Pruitt, L. D., Luxton, D. D., Johnson, K. Patient perceptions of telemental health: systematic review of direct comparisons to in-person psychotherapeutic treatments. *Telemed. E-Health* 2015;21: 652–60.

6. Woodward, K., Kanjo, E., Brown, D. J. et al. Beyond mobile apps: a survey of technologies for mental well-being. *IEEE Trans. Affect. Comput.* 2022;13(3): 1216–35. https://doi.org/10.1109/TAFFC.2020.3015018.

7. Iacobucci, G. Row over Babylon's chatbot shows lack of regulation. *BMJ* 2020;368: m815. https://doi.org/10.1136/bmj.m815.

8. McGinnis, J. M., Williams-Russo, P., Knickman, J. R. The case for more active policy attention to health promotion. *Health Aff. (Millwood)* 2002;21: 78–93.

9. Gray, M. Value based healthcare. *BMJ* 2017;356: j437. https://doi.org/10.1136/bmj.j437.

10. Design Council. The Double Diamond. 2023. Available at: www.designcouncil.org.uk/our-resources/the-double-diamond/ (accessed 20 June 2023).

11. Trebble, T. M., Hansi, N., Hydes, T., Smith, M. A., Baker, M. Process mapping the patient journey: an introduction. *BMJ* 2010;341: c4078.

12. Carpenter, B. Understanding all the barriers service users might face. *Government Digital Service*. 26 March 2019. Available at: https://gds.blog.gov.uk/2019/03/26/understanding-all-the-barriers-service-users-might-face/ (accessed 20 June 2023).

13. Greenhalgh, T., Wherton, J., Papoutsi, C. et al. Beyond adoption: a new framework for theorizing and evaluating nonadoption, abandonment, and challenges to the scale-up, spread, and sustainability of health and care technologies. *J. Med. Internet Res.* 2017;19: e367.

14. Carnegie, D. *How to Win Friends and Influence People*. London: Vermilion. 2006.

15. UK Government. Agile delivery. 2023. Available at: www.gov.uk/service-manual/agile-delivery (accessed 20 June 2023).

16. ICO. Consent. 2023. Available at: https://ico.org.uk/for-organisations/guide-to-data-protection/guide-to-the-general-data-protection-regulation-gdpr/lawful-basis-for-processing/consent/ (accessed 20 June 2023).

17. NHS Digital. Digital Clinical Safety training. 2023. Available at: https://digital.nhs.uk/services/clinical-safety/clinical-risk-management-training (accessed 20 June 2023).

18. NHS Digital. Clinical safety documentation. 2023. Available at: https://digital.nhs.uk/services/clinical-safety/documentation (accessed 20 June 2023).

19. Medicines and Healthcare products Regulatory Agency. 2014, last updated 2023. Medical devices: software applications (apps). Available at: www.gov.uk/government/publications/medical-devices-software-applications-apps (accessed 20 June 2023).

20. NHS England – Transformation Directorate. Digital Technology Assessment Criteria (DTAC). 2023. Available at: www.nhsx.nhs.uk/key-tools-and-info/digital-technology-assessment-criteria-dtac/ (accessed 20 June 2023).

21. NHS Health Research Authority. Is my study research? 2023. Available at: www.hra-decisiontools.org.uk/research/ (accessed 20 June 2023).

22. NHS England. NHS Accelerated Access Collaborative: Embedding research in the NHS. 2023. Available at: www.england.nhs.uk/aac/what-we-do/embedding-research-in-the-nhs/# (accessed 20 June 2023).

23. NHS England. Quality, service improvement and redesign (QSIR) tools. 2023. Available at: www.england.nhs.uk/sustainableimprovement/qsir-programme/qsir-tools/ (accessed 20 June 2023).

24. Killin, L. O. J., Russ, T. C. Surdhar, S. K. et al. Digital Support Platform: a qualitative research study investigating the feasibility of an internet-based, postdiagnostic support platform for families living with dementia. *BMJ Open* 2018;8: e020281. http://dx.doi.org/10.1136/bmjopen-2017-020281.

Note Keeping in the Digital Age
Making Good Use of Electronic Records Systems

Hashim Reza

Psychiatric history taking and its documentation is a core skill that all clinical members of a mental health team need to learn at an early stage of their training. The narrative format has been well established and is followed in all mental health services and sub-specialities. This puts it in contrast with most physical health disciplines and poses unique challenges when attempts have been made to digitise the clinical information. This chapter reviews the background and legacy that needs to be preserved, reviews the lessons learnt over a decade of using Electronic Health Record (EHR) systems and considers approaches that can facilitate the development of standards for note keeping and clinical documentation in digital information systems.

History of Mental Health Records

A cursory look through the case books of mental asylums of the Victorian era shows that a structured format for note keeping had evolved by the end of the nineteenth century. The case books of Bexley Asylum from 1912 reviewed by the author show admission notes of patients written in a structured format with headings that are in use more than a century later. This suggests that the structured format that has been followed by many generations of psychiatrists had been finalised in the first half of the twentieth century. The ubiquitous psychiatric summary that is considered the evidence of a full and proper assessment of a patient is best exemplified in the *Maudsley Handbook of Practical Psychiatry* that most psychiatrists in the UK have been familiar with since the earliest days of their postgraduate training.[1] In an era when most clinical contacts and almost all initial assessments took place in hospital settings, it thus became standard practice that Part 1 of this summary – comprising 13 headings that provided the details of presenting symptoms, past psychiatric history, personal and developmental details and family history – was required to be completed within the first week of admission of a patient and Part 2 – that provided a summary of interventions and treatments during the hospital stay – soon after their discharge from hospital.

In the wake of various policy developments of the 1960s and 1970s that resulted in the closing down of the mental hospitals, integration of mental health services with general hospital and medical services, and transfer of mental healthcare into the community, the format of psychiatric note keeping remained more or less unchanged over the subsequent decades. This could be taken as sufficient evidence that it served the purposes of supporting continuity of care within mental health services but also across different professional disciplines in primary and secondary services in the NHS.

Various headings of different sections of the psychiatric summary have subsequently been adopted into the Standards for the Clinical Structure and Content of Patient Records through extensive collaborative work with professional bodies and medical Royal Colleges led by the Health Informatics Unit of the Royal College of Physicians, London, in 2015.[2] These standards are also the basis of the subsequent work that the Professional Records Standards Body (PRSB) has been leading on.

Professional bodies and regulatory authorities, such as the General Medical Council, UK (GMC),[3] the Royal College of Psychiatrists (RCPsych)[4] and the British Psychological Society (BPS),[5] have produced guidance on record-keeping standards. Such guidance tends to reflect the regulatory authority's objectives of ensuring public safety. Additionally, organisations providing indemnity insurance also have guidance and advisory notes to support professional practice in the case of litigation and disputes about care provision.[6, 7]

The legacy clinical records systems thus comprised mostly handwritten notes that were summarised into reports and clinic letters by medical secretaries that were the backbone of every clinical team. These reports and letters provided snapshots of different episodes of care in a longitudinal care record. They also supported communications and workflows within a multi-disciplinary team and with the primary care services as well as other secondary care services in case it became necessary to refer a patient elsewhere.

A significant point that deserves highlighting is that clinical records have always had the primary objective of supporting clinical care. This key observation was reiterated repeatedly in policy documents and directives regarding clinical records as the NHS services were being developed in the early 1950s. However, since the increase in managerialism that started with the NHS reforms of the 1980s, the imperatives of monitoring the activities in the mental health service and associated costs, euphemistically referred to as productivity, have constantly added to the reporting requirements. Many of these practices had started well before the advent of the EHRs but the clinical staff had not been burdened with the responsibility of collecting this information that has doubtful relevance to direct clinical care.

It also is worth noting that doctors have been complaining about the burden of note keeping from as early as 1956.[8] Innovative approaches were adopted in the 1980s to organise bulky, unmanageable and chaotic records into a bulky but manageable and organised record using the new Aberdeen Medical Record.[9, 10]

Electronic Health Records

As computers became widely available in the late 1990s, attempts were made in many mental health services to standardise assessments and care planning using templates in Microsoft Word. A major driver for this was the Care Programme Approach (CPA) implemented in the Standards for the Clinical Structure and Content of Patient Records of mental health services in England as part of the Health of the Nation strategy in the 1990s.[11] These templates served as the starting point a decade or so later for configuring computerised care records services that were implemented through the National Programme for IT in 2005–12.[12, 13]

Some innovative mental health trusts had implemented Health Information Systems (HIS) in the 1990s based on database systems that were primarily used by hospital managers and admin staff in the clinical teams for managing appointments and scheduling of care such as hospital admissions and detentions under the Mental Health Act. Although these systems were not meant for clinical note keeping, they can be considered a bridge between the traditional paper-based clinical records and patient management systems.

By the time the National Programme for IT (NPfIT) was launched in 2002,* mental health services in the UK were using a combination of systems: scheduling and activity data in the HIS or similar patient information management systems along with paper-based clinical records, word-processed documents that were mostly hospital discharge summaries, clinical letters, reports of specialised assessments and documents related to the CPA process such as care plans, risk assessments, and crisis and contingency plans.[14, 15] The funding available through NPfIT enabled a large number of mental health trusts to adopt EHRs though some trusts had also implemented EHRs independently around the same time. By the time NPfIT was wound down in 2015, there were at least four commercial suppliers that had their EHRs implemented in around 60% of mental health trusts in England: Servelec Healthcare RiO, Advanced Carenotes, TPP SystmOne and Civica Paris. Mental health services in Scotland, Wales and Northern Ireland had their own programmes for digitising their services, often sharing a system with physical health due to their territorial health board structure.

Strengths and weaknesses of these EHR systems have been reviewed and reported extensively.[16] They are summarised in Box 3.1. After nearly 15 years of their use in the majority of mental health services in the UK, the primary benefit is the ready accessibility of clinical information to all those who need access for legitimate reasons from multiple sites at all times. This greatly facilitates timely delivery of care. Over the past few years, many regions in the UK have also developed local shared care record services, further supporting care provision and avoiding delays.

Despite variation in the design and functions of different clinical information systems provided by commercial suppliers, the basic structure of the EHRs is essentially similar. These systems have been designed primarily to support scheduling of care – such as bed management and clinic bookings – and capture data that was considered necessary to monitor CPA activity including referrals, admissions, discharges, length of stay in the

---

Box 3.1 Electronic Health Records – benefits and burdens

Benefits

Clinical notes are legible and accessible to multiple staff working from different sites at the same time.
    Real-time (and near real-time) monitoring of patients and caseloads possible when clinical information is coded.
    Research supported by population-level datasets.

Burdens

Little more than electronic filing cabinets.
    Too many 'clicks' to get to the relevant page/screen in the case records.
    Critical information ('signal') at risk of being lost in vast amounts of free text ('noise').
    Multiple copies of the same information recorded in different sections of the care records at different times create conflicts and patient safety risks.

---

* NPfIT is discussed in detail in Chapter 1.

caseload of a clinical team, detentions under the Mental Health Act and so on. The EHRs have tried to replicate the traditional structure of clinical notes in psychiatry through adding to the core database clinical document functions of variable sophistication based mostly on free-text entries that are generally referred to as 'forms'.

Forms are an artefact of paper-based systems: a vehicle to store and share information. Our attempts to replicate these on screen in electronic systems has taken away the flexibility that the pen–paper interface provides. Instead, time needed to complete records has increased many-fold and frequently the information recorded in different forms in the same set of records adds unresolved contradictions within the information.

When presenting to the Informatics Conference at the Royal College of Psychiatrists on 26 September 2018, Dr Nicola Byrne, in her role then as Chief Clinical Information Officer at the South London and Maudsley NHS Foundation Trust, summarised this unintended consequence of digital systems: 'In more than 15 years of using these systems, no one has ever asked to take anything away. We have only ever asked to add more and more. Every time a new problem comes up, people think if we just build a box to tick for it, then that's problem solved. Furthermore, subject matter experts leading on an issue, often only think about their "thing" without seeing the bigger picture.' This has resulted in creating more and more forms that yet fail to provide a reliable summary of the care issues that a patient has at a given time.

The problem gets further compounded when most information is noted in free text. There still is a widespread practice of dictating letters and reports that are then scanned back into the EHR of the patient. This vast amount of clinical information in free text, thus uncoded, or in scanned documents that are hard to view, browse or read and impossible to search has created a 'dark clinical record', a term first used by Dr Marcus Baw, a GP leader in health informatics (copied from exchanges in the Digital Health CCIO Network). As clinical records get bigger, this dark record is a source of significant risk.

Most importantly, despite considerable efforts over a decade and more, only a few mental health services in England have implemented electronic prescribing and medicines administration systems (ePMA), whilst the Hospital Electronic Prescribing and Medicine Administration (HEPMA) programme has been rolled out in Scotland. In the vast majority of mental health services, prescribing and medicines management has continued through paper-based medicines charts. The ePMA systems that have been implemented struggle to support the routine use of medicines that are unique to psychiatric practice.

Current Challenges

Mediocre usability of EHR systems implemented in mental health services emerged as a theme in the earliest reports that were formally commissioned for the evaluation of the NPfIT. Over the subsequent years, several attempts have been made to conduct national usability surveys with a view to identify what works well and where improvements are needed in the systems. The results have, however, been shared and reviewed only in closed groups of those in formal leadership roles at different organisations.

The first attempt was in 2012 through a small number of collaborating NHS trusts that used different configurations of the same electronic system, namely Servelec RiO (personal communication). In 2016, NHS England, the Chief Clinical Information Officer Leaders Network and Digital Health Intelligence launched the first national Clinical Systems Usability Survey (cSUS) to assess all the main electronic patient record and clinical systems in use across the NHS.[17] The Royal College of Psychiatrists supported this survey and publicised it to all its members. The aim of the survey was to improve the availability of standardised, trustworthy data that can better inform NHS purchasing decisions and encourage the health IT industry to make improvements in their software by asking front-line clinical staff to rate the software they used. More than 1,300 clinicians provided feedback on the survey, with many clinicians giving the software they use an overall rating of 'OK'. The results, however, did not get published though were presented to the CCIO Summer School in 2016, essentially showing that none of the EHRs in use met the average industry standards and that there were considerable variations in user experience at different organisations for the same EHR system determined by local factors.

NHSX conducted a national survey of EHR usability in August 2021.[18] The survey was developed in partnership with an international research agency called KLAS. Several thousand frontline staff responded to the survey but the results have again not been published but shared as feedback to participating NHS Trusts.

Poor user experience of EHRs currently available is proving costly in time for all clinical and professional staff. The dependency on a computer keyboard as the main interface between the user and the EHR has slowed down the clinical work whilst interfering adversely with clinician–patient interaction. Inordinate time is taken in both searching for information that is essential to support a clinical consultation and when noting clinical findings and observations. Technical solutions such as speech recognition could be one approach to replace the support that had previously been provided by medical secretaries, but such solutions pose their unique challenges that have created hurdles in their adoption.

Related issues are the workflows and scheduling that the current EHRs handle badly. These were also traditionally managed by medical secretaries. There is a need to add functions or link additional solutions to EHRs to reduce the burden on the clinical staff to free up their time for direct care.

There is also the need for existing information in the EHR to be available readily in a structured and organised format that supports the delivery of care. The information on assessments, their conclusions and care needs, care plan actions and their scheduling currently sit in silos in EHRs. If this information can be linked better to create a coherent clinical picture, that could greatly enhance the quality of care and reduce the margin of errors.

The use of EHRs has expanded the meaning of clinical record beyond the traditional psychiatric summary, assessment reports, clinic letters and associated notes of clinical observations. With the adoption of digital information systems in hospital and community pharmacies, pathology laboratories, radiology and imaging services, and different specialist services, the nature of a complete and accurate clinical record is now considerably wider. There have also been efforts to link up clinical records with the local authority social care teams' datasets to create a holistic picture of the social and healthcare needs of a citizen. The Local Health and Care Record Exemplars initiative by NHS England in 2018 provided a significant resource in this regard.[19] The shared care records services that have been implemented in many regions of England and in Northern Ireland provide this function through read-only access with the challenge of there being no single truth in the data. Considerable challenges continue regarding the provenance of data and related information, its accuracy and timeliness that can ensure safe delivery of care without delays.

For years, staff working in the health and social care services have looked towards statutory bodies such as NHS Digital for developing standards that address the aforementioned challenges. The technical teams in these organisations in turn have looked towards the professional bodies to provide guidance. Whilst the Royal College of Psychiatrists produced detailed guidance for the general public regarding EHRs that had been available on their website for a few years until a recent update of the website, guidance on standards of note keeping in these systems for the College members remains lacking. Review of guidance on the BPS website discusses issues of information governance without addressing how note keeping needs to change in the era of EHRs.[5]

Future State

Psychiatry remains a clinical discipline primarily despite the breakthroughs in brain sciences during the closing decades of the last century. The aetiology of mental disorders mostly remains undetermined and the mechanisms of how these disorders manifest are not adequately explained by the scientific models. It remains a distant goal that assessment and monitoring of mental health issues can be based on easily coded clinical information, which in turn can drive algorithms linked with clinical decision support systems that get regularly updated by an emerging evidence base. Patient narrative therefore maintains the primary importance it has had thus far. It is likely to continue as the fundamental plank in clinical methods for many years to come.

As the very first step, mental health services and informatics leaders need to move beyond the concept of forms and need to consider instead the information sets/subsets that are contained in these forms. Whereas traditionally a clinic letter or hospital discharge summary inevitably communicated these information sets bundled together, as we now have the ability to record and access information readily, some subsets of information need updating in an information system only if the information contained therein changes. However, the challenge is to provide such information readily for the purpose of verification without it being buried deep in the system, requiring complex steps or multiple 'clicks' to access it.

There is then a need to replicate the traditional structure of psychiatric summary in its various sections and headings to create a structured set of notes that starts curtailing the use of free text. There must be an emphasis on using standard clinical terms when noting presenting complaints, history of these presenting complaints, personal and developmental history, family history and previous medical and psychiatric history, and the mental state examination. For example, if the presence or absence of diurnal variation in mood or early morning wakening is mentioned in a note entry along with the usual list of depressive symptoms, some EHRs can match these standard terms to international coding systems. Similarly, using the standard phenomenological terms to describe a specific thought disorder or auditory verbal hallucinations in a patient suffering with psychosis can then be matched to codes in international glossaries.

Writing a formulation or clinical summary that succinctly captures the bio-psycho-social issues impacting on a patient's condition at a given time has always been considered the high point of clinical competence in mental health. There is a great need to revive this skill, as has been highlighted in a recent paper by the Royal College of Psychiatrists (the Occasional Papers are documents for the members of RCPsych and may not be readily accessible to the general public).[20] It can be argued that such a formulation needs to be the 'landing page' in the electronic care record of a patient in every mental health service.

The standard glossaries of structured clinical terms need an information/data model to determine how the clinical information is mapped and stored in the EHR. If, as the very minimum, all the key elements of information in a formulation can be coded, this can enable clinical decision support tools to support workflows and monitor care against the guidelines and professional standards.

Electronic systems are better able to support creation of patient narrative through dialogue. At the very minimum, patients should be able to write their personal and developmental history. It has been traditional in many children and adolescent mental health services (CAMHS) that the patient and their carers were invited to provide their personal and developmental details in advance of their first assessment by the clinical team. Technology now enables this practice to be replicated in the EHRs. Some mental health services have started providing EHR access to patients that is currently read-only. This needs to be enhanced and made a universal standard for all EHR systems that patients are able to write their narrative and comment on what healthcare staff write in their notes. Patients should thus be able to grow the records through their ability to offer critiques and alternative explanations. Merely allowing patients to peruse their records is not a sufficient objective to aim for.

Finally, the EHRs have not just replaced the traditional case notes and clinical records on paper but have also replaced some of the routine practices in care management and clinical workflows that remain rudimentary and erratic, requiring considerable improvement and refinement. As this work gets pursued, there is a great risk that the focus shifts away from the central place that the clinical narrative has in the clinical records. There is a need to ensure that enhancements to EHR systems are not at the cost of compromising the clinical narrative and ready access to the core clinical issues noted in the records. This has implications not just for design and configuration of the systems but for training of the staff using these systems to ensure their competencies.

Conclusions

The mental health clinical record has evolved through a long journey and its structure has been stable for decades. Until the scientific basis of mental disorders is understood at an aetiological level, the current format of case notes needs to be replicated in EHRs but the use of free text needs to be curtailed. Better design of EHRs and increased use of standard clinical terms can enhance the ability to code information in the EHRs. This in turn can support adoption of technical solutions that better manage workflows and provide clinical decision support to reduce variation in care and ensure a higher quality of care.

Professional bodies need to develop guidance for their members and the competencies impacting on use of EHRs need to be part of training curricula and evaluations.

Further reading

Gillum, R. F. From papyrus to the electronic tablet: a brief history of the clinical medical record with lessons for the digital age. *Am J. Med.* 2013;126: 853–7 http://dx.doi.org/10.1016/j.amjmed.2013.03.024.

Greenhalgh, T., Keen, J. England's national programme for IT. *Br. Med. J.* 2013;346: 4130. https://doi.org/10.1136/bmj.f4130.

Mann, R., Williams, J. Standards in medical record keeping. *Clin. Med.* 2003;3(4): 329–32.

Murphy, J. W., Choi, J. M., Cadeiras, M. The role of clinical records in narrative medicine: a discourse of message. *Perm. J.* 2017;20(2): 103–8.

Professional Records Standards Body. Available at: https://theprsb.org/ (accessed 20 June 2023).

Richardson J., McDonald J. Digitally enabled patients, professionals and providers: making the case for an electronic health record in

mental health services. *BJPsych Bull.* 2016;40 (5): 277–80.

Tait, I. History of our records. *Br. Med. J.* 1981;282: 702–4.

Turner, J., Hayward, R., Angel, K. et al. The history of mental health services in modern England: practitioner memories and the direction of future research. *Med. Hist.* 2015;59(4): 599–624.

References

1. Owen, G., Wessely, S., Murray, R. *The Maudsley Handbook of Practical Psychiatry.* 6th ed. Oxford: Oxford University Press. 2014.

2. Royal College of Physicians. *Standards for the Clinical Structure and Content of Patient Records.* 2015. Available at: www.rcplondon.ac.uk/projects/outputs/standards-clinical-structure-and-content-patient-records (accessed 20 June 2023).

3. General Medical Council, UK. Good medical practice. Available at: www.gmc-uk.org/-/media/documents/good-medical-practice—english-20200128_pdf-51527435.pdf (accessed 20 June 2023).

4. Royal College of Psychiatrists. *Good Psychiatric Practice.* 3rd ed. College Report CR154, p. 12. 2009. Available at: www.rcpsych.ac.uk/docs/default-source/improving-care/better-mh-policy/college-reports/college-report-cr154.pdf?sfvrsn=e196928b_2 (accessed 20 June 2023).

5. British Psychological Society. *Electronic Records Guidance.* 2019. Available at: https://explore.bps.org.uk/content/report-guideline/bpsrep.2019.rep125 (accessed 20 June 2023).

6. Medical Protection Society. Record-keeping. 2018. Available at: www.medicalprotection.org/uk/articles/record-keeping-uk (accessed 20 June 2023).

7. Medical Defence Union. Effective record keeping. 2021. www.themdu.com/guidance-and-advice/guides/effective-record-keeping (accessed 20 June 2023).

8. Fry, J., Blake, P. Keeping of records in general practice. *Br. Med. J.* 1956;1 (suppl 2681): 339–341.

9. Wilson, L. A., Petrie, J. C., Dawson, A. A., Marron, A. C. A new Aberdeen Medical Record. *Br. Med. J.* 1978;2(6134): 414–15.

10. Rix, K. J. B., McNally, B., Johnson, M. A psychiatric version of the New Aberdeen Medical Record. *Bull. R. Coll. Psychiatrists* 1983; 7(11): 201–2.

11. Department of Health. *The Care Programme Approach for People with a Mental Illness, Referred to Specialist Psychiatric Services.* Joint Health/Social Services Circular HC(90) 23/LASSL(90)11. 1990.

12. eHealth Insider. Six London trusts get RiO for mental health. 3 October 2007. Available at: www.digitalhealth.net/2007/10/six-london-trusts-get-rio-for-mental-health/ (accessed 20 June 2023).

13. eHealth Insider. Its name is RiO. 3 December 2008. Available at: www.digitalhealth.net/2008/12/its-name-is-rio/

14. Hunt, J. The M: drive project. *Br. J. Healthc. Comput. Inform. Manage.* 2002;19: 20–2.

15. Treloar, A., Hunt, J. Clinically useful electronic patient record. *Psychiatr. Bull.* 2002; 226(8): 315. https://doi.org/10.1192/pb.26.8.315-b.

16. Takian, A., Sheikh, A., Barber, N. We are bitter, but we are better off: case study of the implementation of an electronic health record system into a mental health hospital in England. *BMC Health Serv. Res.* 2012;12: 484. https://doi.org/10.1186/1472-6963-12-484.

17. Digital Health Intelligence. CSUS: big differences in usability of clinical software. 2 June 2016. Available at: www .digitalhealth.net/2016/06/csus-big-differences-in-usability-of-clinical-software/ (accessed 20 June 2023).

18. Digital Health Intelligence. NHSX launches national survey to better understand EPR usability. 12 August 2021. Available at: www.digitalhealth.net/2021/08/nhsx-launches-national-survey-to-better-understand-epr-usability/ (accessed 20 June 2023).

19. NHS England. *Local Health and Care Records Exemplars*. 2018. Available at: www .england.nhs.uk/publication/local-health-and-care-record-exemplars/ (accessed 20 June 2023).

20. Royal College of Psychiatrists. Using formulation in general psychiatric care: good practice. OP103. January 2017. Available at: www.rcpsych.ac.uk/docs/default-source/files-for-college-members/occasional-papers/occasional-paper-103.pdf?sfvrsn=4255f943_2 (accessed 20 June 2023).

Big Data
The New Epidemiology

Lucy Stirland, Tom Russ and Tom Foley

Introduction

The term 'big data' has been used increasingly in healthcare research in the first two decades of the twenty-first century. Most definitions focus on its characteristics, namely volume, variety and velocity, and other attributes have been identified including veracity, variability and value. There is no consensus on the volume that is classed as 'big'. This is summarised in Figure 4.1. It is clear that big data reflects advances in information technology and the ability to store, securely access, manage and analyse large-volume datasets.[1]

One approach to defining size is that big data requires high-powered storage and analytic methods.[2] 'Big data' is also used by technology companies to refer to information gathered about the public, often personal in nature or relating to their use of devices or platforms. In any setting, the large size can come from the breadth of a dataset (how many people's data are included), its depth (the number of variables per person) or both.

Data science can be understood as the process of generating new knowledge from real-world high-volume datasets, using statistics and data analysis methodology.[3]

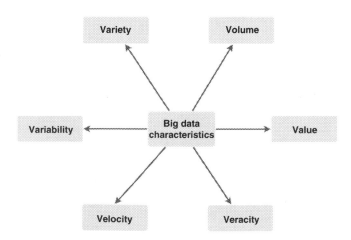

Figure 4.1 Attributes of 'big data'

Data Sources

Data for scientific use can come from routinely collected health records, observational research studies, trials and the emerging area of personal technology, including smartphone applications, social media and wearables.

Healthcare

Each individual interacting with a healthcare system generates substantial amounts of data which are used for their own care; this data can additionally be used for research purposes, subject to consent and appropriate regulatory safeguards. In England, over 100 national data collections cover all aspects of the NHS. The first of these was Hospital Episode Statistics, which has been collected by NHS Digital and its predecessor organisations since 1989. Equivalents in other nations are the Scottish Morbidity Record, which has been available since 1981, and the Patient Episode Database in Wales since 1991. In Northern Ireland, the Honest Broker Service for Health and Social Care collates and securely shares individual-level linked data across the integrated health and social care system.

Structured data about every patient treated in acute hospitals was originally extracted by an army of clinical coders who reviewed paper notes. This data was submitted on a monthly basis and made available for planning, policymaking and research. The Mental Health Services Data Set and the Improving Access to Psychological Therapies Data Set contain clinical and administrative data on the interactions of patients with secondary care mental health services and psychological services, respectively.

Richer clinical data can be found in Electronic Health Records, although such records are often not interoperable between providers. In mental health in particular, data is often held as unstructured free text, for example, clinical letters.

Whilst health services have been routinely collecting this data and publishing summary statistics for many years, the Covid-19 pandemic raised the public profile of day-to-day routine data reporting.

Research

Large, repeated population surveys, such as the Health Survey for England and the Scottish Health Survey, are conducted at regular intervals and contain some information on mental health. More detail is gathered by the Adult Psychiatric Morbidity Survey and the Mental Health of Children and Young People Survey. Such surveys provide detailed regional snapshots of the prevalence of mental health conditions and life experiences. Data on the participants in these surveys can be linked to health service usage data within the national data collections mentioned above, in order to provide additional prognostic information.

Whilst few mental health disorders are the result of single genetic mutations, genome-wide association studies have identified associations between many mental health disorders and a range of common genetic variants. Inexpensive genotyping microarrays can provide information on millions of common variants and are likely to have a larger clinical role in the future.

Polygenic risk scores could be calculated to give an indication of likelihood of individual disorders, as well as prognosis, efficacy of treatments and likelihood of side effects.

Personal Technology

Data is also generated outside the healthcare system. Consumer products containing sensors capable of recording location, movement, light and an increasing range of digital and physiological biomarkers are becoming more popular and affordable.

Modern smartphones contain an array of sensors and interaction with the phone itself can provide clues to a person's mental state. Taps, finger movements, unlocks, notifications, charges, app usage, call and SMS frequency, as well as calendar data can be collected.

In current practice, a patient is often asked to report to a clinician on variations in their mental state that occurred weeks, months or even years ago. This may or may not be accurately recorded in the Electronic Health Record. Ecological momentary assessment is an approach that aims to record a person's behaviour and experiences in real time in their natural environment. Smartphones offer the opportunity for regular or event-based experience sampling and recording of patient-reported outcomes and apps already exist to monitor mental health symptoms and predict relapse.[4] The Covid Symptoms Study has collected daily updates from over 4.6 million volunteers through a smartphone app, and it publishes research illustrating the powerful potential of this form of data collection.[5]

Novel sources of data are becoming available to health and commercial researchers. Research using Google Trends data has also been used to examine responses to celebrity suicides as well as infectious diseases.[6] Ingestible sensors have been developed that can monitor whether a patient is taking their medication and skin-worn sensors that can detect stress-related hormones are under development. Many people place rich phenotypic data on social media and researchers have already explored how this could be harnessed. Each data source has pros and cons and in many areas the ethics and clinical utility of using such data has not been established.

Using Routinely Collected Data in Psychiatry

Routinely collected data can be harnessed to improve psychiatric care and outcomes through surveillance, prediction and quality improvement and to inform policy.

Surveillance systems use data to identify changes in the distribution of health-related phenomena. The Covid-19 pandemic has highlighted the importance of infectious disease surveillance, but the same approach can be applied to other issues such as suicide rates or adverse reactions to medications.

Pattern recognition, based on historical data, can be used to infer what might happen in the future, for example, what treatment might be effective given a particular set of circumstances or what high-risk or high-cost events are likely to occur.

Like screening tools, predictive models generate true positives, true negatives, false positives and false negatives and these can all be associated with harm. This must be considered in the development of such models.

Quality improvement methods are generally driven by data. For example, data containing outcome or process measures can be used to benchmark teams, organisations, regions or entire countries. Positive deviance involves identifying groups that are performing particularly well, studying them to understand why they perform well and then working with other groups to share the good practice.

Large-volume healthcare data is valuable for policymaking and public health. The trends of specific diagnoses or clinical presentations can be tracked through coded records, allowing service planning and informing public health interventions. Data can also be used to monitor the impact of a policy's implementation.[7] Summary data is often publicly available online through the Office for National Statistics and Scottish Public Health Observatory, for example, on suicide rates and related demographics.

Prescribing records can be particularly enlightening in psychiatry, as seen in regular media attention to published increasing rates of antidepressant prescription. This is especially useful when drugs are only used for one indication, for example, with the drugs for dementia. A Scottish research study linked prescribing data with hospital diagnoses amongst people with bipolar disorder and found a decrease in the prescription of lithium between 2009 and 2016, highlighting a real-world deviation from best practice guidelines.[8]

Harnessing routine data in this way has the major strength of including people who are often missed or intentionally excluded from cohort studies and trials. This is pertinent in psychiatry where patients may be under-represented in traditional research because of severe mental illness, multimorbidity or lacking capacity due to cognitive impairment or intellectual disability. An example of this is The Health Improvement Network, which uses GP data from over 3.7 million patients to create a sample representative of the UK population. A 2015 study used this database to ascertain that people with intellectual disability received a disproportionately high number of psychotropic prescriptions.[9]

Research

Routinely collected data can support traditional research. The NHS Digital DigiTrials service uses the national data collections in England to assist researchers planning clinical trials. It can inform them on whether there are enough patients in a region who meet proposed inclusion criteria, for example, how many patients have a particular condition. It can then identify potential participants and contact them on behalf of the researchers.

Once enrolled in the trial, DigiTrials can enable low-cost and convenient long-term follow-up by reporting on health service usage over time (e.g. new diagnoses and treatments).

Healthcare data can also be used directly for research. Whilst coded diagnoses and population-level summary statistics are useful for understanding larger questions, the majority of clinical notes in psychiatry comprise free-text entries and pose limitations for quantitative research. The South London and Maudsley NHS Foundation Trust Biomedical Research Centre Case Register and its Clinical Record Interactive Search (CRIS) hold over 250,000 linked patient records for research. Their innovative methods include the application of natural language processing techniques, which convert free text into structured tables. Introducing these techniques in this dataset have provided information on cognitive function, education, social care and smoking status (see Box 4.1).[11]

Box 4.1 Example of successful use of routine data in research

- Cholinesterase inhibitors had been found in randomised controlled trials (RCTs) to temporarily slow cognitive decline in people with Alzheimer's dementia.
- RCTs often exclude people with multimorbidity or advanced illness, potentially comprising the majority of people with dementia. Real-world evidence was needed.
- A 2014 observational study extracted text from the health records of 2,460 patients prescribed these drugs in London, UK, and found similar effects to the trials.
- This study allowed larger sample sizes, broader inclusion criteria and longer follow-up than the RCTs.[10]

Aside from routine healthcare data, other large-volume datasets can come from specifically designed observational studies, either retrospective or prospective. UK Biobank is a population-based cohort study of over 500,000 people aged 40–69 years at recruitment. Participants underwent detailed measurements including genetic testing and neuroimaging, as well as cognitive testing and mental health questionnaires. They have regular follow-up and, if consented, their linked NHS data is available to researchers.[12]

Challenges and Limitations

Data Capture

Data can be captured in many ways: through sensors or as a by-product of the use of other systems such as smartphones. Some of the most useful data is entered into Electronic Health Records, by clinicians or patients. Highly structured input fields can be used to capture structured data or natural language processing (NLP) can be used to make sense of free text. Some providers still rely on clinical coders to extract data from handwritten notes. These coders are trained but are not members of the treating medical team, leading to potential discrepancies between the clinical impression and the coded diagnosis. Structured data, such as genomic or pathology results, can be captured directly from labs, if standards are agreed.

Findings from any dataset are limited to the participants represented within that dataset. This is most obvious in research studies where selection bias leads to disproportionate representation of certain socioeconomic and ethnic groups. This phenomenon also occurs in routinely collected healthcare data; it is only available from patients who access healthcare. In settings with universal healthcare, this is less of a prominent issue but still leads to the under-representation of the hardest-to-reach groups, risking perpetuating health inequalities.

Data Quality and Provenance

If data is incomplete, inaccurate or out of date, then the insights drawn from it may not be accurate. Data is often collated from multiple sources and may have been processed and altered by multiple parties. Data provenance is the process of understanding where data has come from and what changes have been made to it.

The quality of the underlying data can vary for many reasons. Some data-quality checks, such as coverage, completeness and validity, can be automated, as with NHS Digital's Data Quality Maturity Index; however, a deeper understanding of quality requires an understanding of the clinical domain and collection process. Poor-quality data will lead to poor-quality data analysis.

Another limitation of administrative healthcare data is that it often lacks detail on social determinants of health. Ethnicity is poorly recorded and there are rarely standardised variables on housing situation, for example. This can be addressed by careful text mining where free-text entries are available, or by triangulating with smaller datasets from tailored cohort studies.[13] There are also opportunities in the future for further linkage with social care, education and criminal justice system data. Academic clinicians play a valuable role in designing research that answers clinically meaningful questions, including understanding specific relevant variables.

There is a need for honesty about the limitations within a dataset and not to use the conclusions of any analysis inappropriately. Epidemiological research findings, for example, should be communicated transparently, with clear statements that observational findings cannot imply causality.

Data Storage

Data can be stored either in local servers or remotely in the cloud. Local servers have the advantage of speed of access and the reassurance that security is locally controlled. The cloud, however, allows instantaneous online backups and continuous software updates.

It might seem like the Electronic Health Record could be used as a repository for data collected from many sources; however, issues around performance, access and interoperability have limited this. Many providers create a data warehouse to hold data from multiple sources, which can then be used for non-clinical purposes. Other platforms have emerged to manage data flowing from outside the clinic and between multiple organisations.

When sharing data between more than one organisation, it can be stored and accessed through centralised or distributed networks. In a centralised network, the data is uploaded to a central repository, from which it can then be accessed. Hospital Episode Statistics data from the English NHS is an example of this approach.

The alternative is a distributed network that leaves each organisation in control of its own protected data. The US Food and Drug Administration (FDA) Mini-Sentinel programme (an active surveillance system for monitoring the safety of FDA-regulated medical products) is an example.[14] Queries are sent to each node (organisation) in the network. They each return results (often aggregated) in an agreed common data model to a coordinating centre.

The centralised model simplifies access to data as only one location needs to be queried; however, the distributed model overcomes many privacy issues and the participating organisations can maintain operational control of their data.

Obstacles to Data Access

Healthcare data is highly personal and sensitive. Keeping it safe from inappropriate access is critical to maintaining trust in its continued collection. Data must be obtained, held, used and shared within a robust and ethical information governance framework. In the UK, information governance is underpinned by the General Data Protection Regulation (GDPR), which is a European Union regulation that has been passed into UK law by the Data Protection Act 2018.[15]

Despite this common legal framework, different data custodians, within and between countries, implement access rules differently. This can lead to significant confusion and delay for those wishing to access data for legitimate uses. The framework also restricts the transfer of data outside the European Economic Area, which may limit opportunities for the globalisation of healthcare.

Large projects that link and share NHS data must be carefully handled to avoid damaging public trust. NHS England's care.data project aimed to link NHS hospital and general practice records, but was abandoned in 2016 after ethical concerns around privacy, data sharing and commercial involvement. The planned launch of the General Practice Data for Planning and Research system was also disrupted in 2021 after criticism about its transparency, reflecting a lack of public trust. There is perhaps increasing discomfort at the idea that technology companies may share or sell data on purchasing patterns. Despite this, there is evidence that the public generally supports linking health data and its analysis by academics and health researchers, as long as this is appropriately conducted and there is no private sector involvement.[16] Whilst the public generally accepts technology and social media companies using their internet use data, often for targeted advertising, health data is perhaps seen as more personal and therefore less appropriate for sharing.

Data Analytics

Once data has been collected and access has been granted – all of which is rarely as straightforward as it could be – it is necessary to analyse the data to draw conclusions. This aspect of data science can range from relatively trivial statistical models summarising the prevalence of a particular condition to complex longitudinal models. However sophisticated the analyses, there is a requirement to be critical of the quality of the data, especially if it was collected for another purpose, for instance routine healthcare. Flaws in how the data was collected or recorded could greatly influence the conclusions drawn from analyses of the data. However, there is a balance to be struck between the size or representativeness of a dataset and the depth or quality of the data recorded about each person included.

When analysing big data, it is important to predefine significance tests that are appropriate to the size of the dataset and number of tests performed. A p-value is the likelihood of obtaining the present results if the null hypothesis is true. Using a p-value cut-off of 0.05 in a large dataset would allow a small effect size to be considered statistically significant. By its definition, 1 in 20 tests will be a false positive. Research results should therefore be presented with more emphasis on effect sizes and confidence intervals, and interpreted accordingly.[17]

We have alluded to the storage challenges associated with big data. The same could be said about analysing such data. Datasets with half a million rows and hundreds of columns require real computing power to run even simple models and, depending on the complexity of the models run, it can feel like one is back in the early days of computing, having to wait a week for an answer! Increased sophistication in statistical approaches and software is helpful here – for example, the development of Integrated Nested Laplace Approximation (INLA), which can produce essentially the same answer as a week's Markov Chain Monte Carlo (MCMC) simulation in about half an hour – as is readier access to 'supercomputers'. Given the dramatic improvements in computer power in recent history, it is expected that analysing such large datasets will become easier. However, with ever-increasing amounts of data being collected, computer power advancements will need to keep up with increases in dataset size.

Translating Knowledge into Practice

Collecting and analysing data is of no value if the knowledge generated is not then used to improve healthcare. Traditionally, these insights have been published in peer-reviewed journals. Whilst this is a valuable activity, it often takes many years for such insights to influence practice. The Covid-19 pandemic has highlighted how important it is for data and insights to be delivered to the frontline more quickly. This requires the creation of Learning Health Systems in which:

- Patients and the public can use data to make decisions about their health and care, including things like choosing a doctor, changing habits based on research or campaigning for change.
- Health professionals can use data to make better clinical decisions, understand patient groups and identify opportunities to improve services.
- Healthcare providers such as hospitals or GPs can use data to plan services and monitor performance against other similar providers.
- Commissioners/payers can use data to understand the changing needs of the population, and to monitor the impact of their work.
- Central NHS organisations can use data to understand population needs and resource requirements over time. They can also monitor quality of care.
- Research organisations (universities, charities, think tanks and companies) can use data to better understand a disease or condition and develop new treatments. They can also assess the efficacy and cost or benefits of existing interventions or even whole health systems.

Taking a broader view of how data and knowledge will be used necessitates a more complex appraisal of whether big data projects will 'work' and what 'working' means. It is not enough to understand whether it is academically possible to generate the knowledge; it is necessary to consider whether the knowledge will be used and useful within the broader healthcare system. The Non-adoption, Abandonment, Scale-up, Spread and Sustainability (NASSS) Framework provides a guide for assessing whether potential projects will be successful.[18] It considers seven domains:

- The Technology: Will it work technically? Will it need to be integrated with other systems? Will it be usable?
- The Condition: What is the clinical scenario? Does it have complex sociocultural factors or common comorbidities that will affect use?
- The Value Proposition: Is the project worth doing, for each stakeholder?
- The Adopter System: Is the system usable by patients, carers and staff? Does it threaten the professional identity of staff?
- The Organisation: Does the organisation in which the project will be deployed have the capability, slack and readiness for change that will be required?
- The Wider Context: Is the project aligned with broader strategy, policy and regulation?
- Embedding and Adaptation over Time: Will the project be able to evolve over time as the world around it changes?

Not every domain in the NASSS Framework will be relevant to every project. For example, some projects will be non-clinical or not patient facing, but generally, the more complexity in each domain, the more likely the project is to fail. Taking a co-design approach to such projects can be an effective way to mitigate these potential issues early.

Conclusions and Future Perspectives

As the use of big data in psychiatry continues to expand, it is crucial to involve patients and the public in decisions about its development and application. Mental Health Data Science Scotland has published a best practice checklist that was co-produced by researchers and

> **Box 4.2 Key learning points**
>
> - Advances in technology and computing provide opportunities for analysing data on a large scale.
> - Large research studies allow detailed phenotyping across numerous characteristics, including genome-wide association studies.
> - Routinely collected healthcare data can inform public health interventions, policymaking and quality improvement.
> - Healthcare data is also valuable for real-world clinical research.
> - Patient and public involvement is key to guiding future uses of healthcare data.

people with lived experience. This guidance emphasises the need for data to be securely accessible and carefully anonymised and for processes and analyses to be transparent, with participants or patients prioritised throughout.[19]

Data about patients, research participants and the public is already collected, stored and maintained. Academics and policymakers have an obligation to use the data to improve care or for high-quality, meaningful research. Key learning points from this chapter are summarised in Box 4.2.

References

1. Schofield, P. Big data in mental health research: do the *n* s justify the means? Using large data-sets of electronic health records for mental health research. *BJPsych. Bull.* 2017;41: 129–32. https://doi.org/10.1192/pb.bp.116.055053.

2. De Mauro, A., Greco, M., Grimaldi, M. What is Big Data? A consensual definition and a review of key research topics. *AIP Conf. Proc.* 2015; 1644(1): 97–104. https://doi.org/10.13140/2.1.2341.5048.

3. Russ, T. C., Woelbert, E., Davis, K. A. S. et al. How data science can advance mental health research. *Nat. Hum. Behav.* 2019;3: 24–32. https://doi.org/10.1038/s41562-018-0470-9.

4. Eisner, E., Drake R. J., Berry N. et al. Development and long-term acceptability of ExPRESS, a mobile phone app to monitor basic symptoms and early signs of psychosis relapse. *JMIR mHealth uHealth* 2019;7: e11568. https://doi.org/10.2196/11568.

5. Menni, C., Valdes, A. M., Freidin, M. B. et al. Real-time tracking of self-reported symptoms to predict potential COVID-19. *Nat. Med.* 2020;26: 1037–40. https://doi.org/10.1038/s41591-020-0916-2.

6. Ortiz, S. N., Forrest, L. N., Fisher, T. J. et al. Changes in internet suicide search volumes following celebrity suicides. *Cyberpsychol. Behav. Soc. Netw.* 2019;22: 373–80. https://doi.org/10.1089/cyber.2018.0488.

7. Vayena, E., Dzenowagis, J., Brownstein, J. S. et al. Policy implications of big data in the health sector. *Bull. World Health Organ.* 2018; 96(1): 66–8. https://doi.org/10.2471/BLT.17.197426.

8. Lyall, L. M., Penades, N., Smith, D. J. Changes in prescribing for bipolar disorder between 2009 and 2016: national-level data linkage study in Scotland. *Br. J. Psychiatry* 2019;215: 415–21. https://doi.org/10.1192/bjp.2019.16.

9. Sheehan, R., Hassiotis, A., Walters, K. et al. Mental illness, challenging behaviour, and psychotropic drug prescribing in people with intellectual disability: UK population based cohort study. *BMJ* 2015;351: h4326. https://doi.org/10.1136/BMJ.H4326.

10. Perera, G., Khondoker, M., Broadbent, M. et al. Factors associated with response to acetylcholinesterase inhibition in dementia: a cohort study from a secondary

mental health care case register in London. *PLoS One* 2014;9: e109484. https://doi.org/10.1371/journal.pone.0109484.

11. Perera, G., Broadbent, M., Callard, F. et al. Cohort profile of the South London and Maudsley NHS Foundation Trust Biomedical Research Centre (SLaM BRC) Case Register: current status and recent enhancement of an Electronic Mental Health Record-derived data resource. *BMJ Open* 2016;6: 8721. https://doi.org/10.1136/bmjopen-2015.

12. Sudlow, C., Gallacher, J., Allen, N. et al. UK Biobank: an open access resource for identifying the causes of a wide range of complex diseases of middle and old age. *PLoS Med* 2015;12: e1001779. https://doi.org/10.1371/journal.pmed.1001779.

13. Arias De La Torre, J., Ronaldson, A., Valderas, J.M. et al. Diagnostic promiscuity: the use of real-world data to study multimorbidity in mental health. *Br. J. Psychiatry* 2021; 218(5): 237–9. https://doi.org/10.1192/bjp.2020.257.

14. Platt, R., Carnahan, R. M., Brown, J. S. et al. The U.S. Food and Drug Administration's Mini-Sentinel program: status and direction. *Pharmacoepidemiol. Drug Saf.* 2012;21: 1–8. https://doi.org/10.1002/pds.2343.

15. Data Protection Act. United Kingdom Act of Parliament. 2018. Available at: www.legislation.gov.uk/ukpga/2018/12/contents/enacted (accessed 16 June 2023).

16. Aitken, M., McAteer, G., Davidson, S. et al. Public preferences regarding data linkage for health research: a discrete choice experiment. *Int. J. Popul. Data Sci.* 2018;3 (1): 429. https://doi.org/10.23889/ijpds.v3i1.429.

17. Sterne, J. A., Davey Smith, G., Smith, G. D. Sifting the evidence: what's wrong with significance tests? *BMJ* 2001;322: 226–31. https://doi.org/10.1136/BMJ.322.7280.226.

18. Greenhalgh, T., Wherton, J., Papoutsi, C. et al. Beyond adoption: a new framework for theorizing and evaluating nonadoption, abandonment, and challenges to the scale-up, spread, and sustainability of health and care technologies. *J. Med. Internet Res.* 2017;19(11): e8775. https://doi.org/10.2196/jmir.8775.

19. Kirkham, E. J., Iveson, M., Beange, I. et al. *A Stakeholder-Derived, Best Practice Checklist for Mental Health Data Science in the UK.* 2020. Edinburgh: University of Edinburgh. Available at: https://mhdss.ac.uk/best-practice-mental-health-data-science (accessed 27 January 2021).

Artificial Intelligence

Why We Need It and Why We Need to Be Cautious

Lesa S. Wright

This chapter serves as an introduction to the significance of artificial intelligence (AI) in psychiatry.

In 1940, Disney released *Fantasia*, an animated feature film, the last segment of which was entitled 'The Sorcerer's Apprentice',[1] which sums up the cautionary tale of AI. It features Mickey Mouse in the role of a sorcerer's apprentice who is seduced by the promise of magical power.

The grand sorcerer tasks Mickey with hauling buckets of water. Naturally, Mickey finds this work tedious and exhausting and quickly realises that with magic, he could get a mop to do the work for him. This goes wonderfully well until the unintended consequence of multiplying mops that relentlessly fetch water, leading to a flood. Mickey is unable to find the right conjuring to stop the deluge. The day is saved when the grand sorcerer returns to find the disaster and casts the right spell to bring it to an end.

This chapter will cover:

- Key definitions (as listed in Table 5.1).
- The need for and advantages of AI in psychiatry.
- The dangers, risks and pitfalls.
- The mitigations against the problems.
- What does the future hold?
- Summary.

The chapter will seek to inform the reader about key and potentially confusing overlapping concepts. The topic will cover the presence of AI technology and its impact in society and influence on the practice of psychiatry. An overview of the evaluation tools and regulatory landscape is also provided.

The Need for and Advantages of AI in Psychiatry

The terms AI and ML are often used interchangeably. In daily life, ML is widely used as narrow AI, but general AI is not. Much of what is referred to as AI is actually ML. Artificial intelligence can be further divided into narrow or weak AI which is focused on one particular task. It could be argued that ML systems such as those that can detect lung cancer from chest X-rays are a form of weak AI. Following on from weak AI is general or strong AI, which is considered to be human-level intelligence and as of now is not known to exist. Super AI is the third category and surpasses human intelligence – it is sometimes described as being able to carry out computational tasks in days or weeks that would take humans tens of thousands of years.[4]

Table 5.1 Key definitions in artificial intelligence

Artificial Intelligence	Artificial intelligence (AI) is intelligence demonstrated by machines, that is, machines that have some of the qualities that the human mind has, such as the ability to understand language, recognise pictures, solve problems and learn.[2].
Machine Learning	Machine learning (ML) is the process of computers changing the way they carry out tasks by learning from new data, without a human being needed to give instructions in the form of a program.[3] Machine learning is one of many routes to AI.
Training	This is the underlying process in machine learning in which individual data points are given weights depending on their significance in a pattern.
Data	Any unit of information such as text, an image, a sound, a symptom, a physiological/psychological measure and so on.
Training Data	The data utilised to train AI/ML systems to perform a function.
Machine Learning Model	An algorithm which is generated through applying ML to training data and can process new and previously unseen data.
Supervised Learning	Supervised learning requires explicit data that is pre-labelled, that is, each unit of data is labelled with information by humans (or automatically or in collaboration). An example of this would be labelling different statements in a clinical record according to the type of symptoms they are associated with.
Unsupervised Learning	A method of learning that does not require labelled data and often used to elicit groups of patterns such as subgroups of patients with symptoms who meet a particular diagnosis.
Reinforcement Learning	A technique in which a model is built by an ML system through trial and error whilst being rewarded for success.
Artificial Neural Network	An algorithm that behaves in a similar way to biological neurons.
Deep Neural Network	An algorithm that contains many layers of 'neurons' and requires great computational power.
Deep Learning	A form of ML that makes use of deep neural networks.

In daily life, many of our interactions with technology involve using ML products. Most of these are geared towards language-based use. These include search engines, email spam filters, recommendations for music and films in streaming services, posts on social media, predictive text on our mobile devices, smart speaker services like Alexa, facial recognition in photos for social media, self-driving cars and credit application systems.

The words 'hope' and 'hype' are frequently used in connection with the application of AI and ML to healthcare. The great driver of progress in contemporary AI and ML seems to be the promise of wealth and power.[5] Both AI and ML have been seen as solutions to multiple problems in every area of care provision, from assessment and diagnosis to treatment, understanding population health and managing supply chains and administrative systems. Processes that are repeatable and standardisable are very well-suited to automation through AI/ML.

The central idea to ML is presenting data to algorithms capable of learning patterns and then recognising these patterns in previously unseen data. There are three primary methods of learning: supervised, unsupervised and reinforcement learning.

There are a wide range of applications of AI/ML to psychiatry and mental health in general:[6]

- personalising treatment selection;
- prognosticating;
- monitoring for relapse;
- detecting and helping to prevent mental health conditions before they reach clinical-level symptomatology;
- delivering some treatments.

Psychiatry benefits particularly well from digitising medical records but computerisation of medical records does not always lead to an increase in productivity of the staff using them. This is referred to as the productivity paradox.[7] The management of this information with AI/ML could potentially overcome the barrier raised by this paradox.

Natural Language Processing

In psychiatry, the application of ML and AI holds promise due to the global shortage of psychiatrists and other mental health workers.[8] This shortage of health workers also applies to other disciplines. Natural language processing (NLP) is a branch of ML which lends itself well to psychiatry's language-centric process. This is not to be confused with neuro-linguistic programming, a form of therapy not used in psychiatric practice.

The use of NLP is established in the following areas in psychiatry:[9]

1. Psychopathology (i.e. observational studies focusing on mental illnesses);
2. The patient perspective (i.e. patients' thoughts and opinions);
3. Medical records (i.e. safety issues, quality of care and description of treatments);
4. Medical literature (i.e. identification of new scientific information in the literature).

Incredible strides have been made in NLP in recent years, particularly with the launch of Generative Pre-trained Transformer 3 (GPT-3) in 2020 by OpenAI. As a language model, GPT-3 'generates AI-written text that has the potential to be practically indistinguishable from human-written sentences, paragraphs, articles, short stories, dialogue, lyrics, and more'. It can write some very convincing articles.[10].

The most public form of AI/ML intervention in psychiatry, namely chatbots or conversational agents, is facilitated by NLP. In the mental wellbeing sphere, these are well established, taking on the role of 'confidant', and acting as screening tools and gateways to human-led therapeutic interventions. Some chatbots go as far as offering a route to conversation with a dead loved one.[11] In the UK, the most well-known mental health chat apps are Woebot[12] and Wysa.[13]

Chatbots may be purely text messaging or voice-based or incorporated into visual 'avatars'. Army veterans in the United States were more readily disposed to disclosure about PTSD-related symptoms when interacting with a chatbot.[14]

In more specific terms, depression is the most studied of all psychiatric conditions with respect to detection and diagnosis; prognosis, treatment and support; public health; and research and clinical administration.[5] This is in part due to its prevalence but also likely due to the apparent ease of converting well-established manualised therapies such as cognitive behavioural therapy (CBT) to automation. Depression is also the target of significant AI/ML interventions in determining medication selection for depression.[15]

Predicting suicide is a difficult, complicated and emotionally challenging process that requires weighing up of multiple variables. The use of ML could help here where other methods have been of limited utility due to ML's ability to account for multiple variables in the pattern recognition routine screening data that could be used to predict suicide attempts.[16]

Text mining is an approach dealing with discovery, retrieval and extraction of information from a corpus of text combining approaches of linguistics, statistics and computer sciences.[9] Text mining leverages NLP and has been applied to Electronic Health Records to perform tasks such as predicting hospital re admission.[17]

The Dangers, Risks and Pitfalls

The risks inherent in AI/ML are well documented. There are general risks which apply to all AI/ML applications.

Bias is a particular problem. It is the difference between predicted and actual values in AI and ML systems.[18] It is the tendency to make predictions or find patterns in data. The bias originates in the data used to train these systems.

There are different types of bias:[19]

- **Sample bias** occurs when there is insufficient variety in the training data. For example, if training an antidepressant response prediction algorithm on data containing almost only women in the age range 30–40 years.
- **Prejudicial bias** occurs when training data contains information that could skew predictions such as race or gender in a system when making recommendations for detention under the Mental Health Act.
- **Exclusion bias** occurs when data is removed during the preparation process that may be a significant factor such as what may be thought to be outliers.
- **Measurement bias** occurs when the training data may, for example, use one method of measurement such as PHQ-9 but the real-world data uses clinical opinion.

Bias has the potential of increasing health inequalities. For example, in the United States ethnic minorities are less likely to have treatments recommended for them because historically they have not accessed these treatments because of the costs involved.[20]

Mental health services do have a problem with race and gender bias. In the UK in 2016/17 and 2017/18, people from black ethnic minorities were almost twice as likely as most other ethnic groups to be detained under the Mental Health Act.[21] In the United States, African Americans are at least one and a half times more likely to be diagnosed with schizophrenia than Caucasians if unstructured diagnostic interviews are used.[22] Historically, women were often more likely to be diagnosed with borderline personality disorder than men even though epidemiological studies indicate there is unlikely to be a difference in rates.[23] The effects of these biases will only be multiplied by using systems that are trained on data containing them without appropriate correction.

An area of great interest is the application of facial recognition to determine emotional states. It creates opportunities in allowing 'holistic assessment' or monitoring of mental state. It is based on the idea that across cultures, six emotional states are consistent.[24]

Although emotion recognition has some real value, for example, in measuring distress in patients with cancer,[25] there are problems. Unfortunately, the datasets used for most emotion recognition system are largely discredited as being unrepresentative and artificial due to the conditions under which images are captured. For example, smiling subjects are assumed to be happy yet most people understand that a smile does not necessarily indicate happiness. There are multiple examples of how facial recognition is actively misused despite the dangers being known. A well-cited study demonstrates that error rates in commercial facial recognition systems can reach 34.7% in darker-skinned females vs 0.8% in lighter-skinned males.[26] As a result of controversy, IBM appeared to scale back its facial recognition services and Microsoft withdrew the largest facial recognition dataset.[27, 28]

If used correctly, facial expression can be used as novel method of diagnosis, as in diagnosing Parkinson's disease through facial expression recognition.[29]

People often do not say what they mean, mean what they say or look how they feel. Affective privacy allows people to make a choice about whether or not to expose their internal state.

There are some significant instructive tales in the deployment of ML tools that, whilst intended to serve some social good, instead resulted in causing harm.

In 2014, the charity Samaritans launched a Twitter app called Radar which 'enabled users to monitor the accounts of their friends for distressing messages'. It was criticised for collecting and highlighting sensitive information about emotional and mental health.[30]

In 2016, Microsoft's 'Tay' was a Twitter chatbot aimed at 18–24-year-olds. Within 24 hours of launch it had learnt from real Twitter users and began to 'tweet wildly inappropriate and reprehensible words and images'. It was taken offline.[31]

Liability in healthcare is a particularly challenging issue. When using an AI decision support tool, who will be held accountable if things go wrong? Is it the human clinician, their employer, the AI system or the AI developer? There are implications for whether clinicians trust AI systems and if patients trust clinicians with AI systems. The use of an AI that fails to perform as expected can lead to claims for property damage, personal injury, professional liability, reputational damage, medical malpractice and cyber risks.[32]

The GPT-3 language model uses deep learning to produce human-like text.[33] It inspires and frightens in equal measure due to the ability to generate text that looks like it has been written by a person with simply a word or sentence as a prompt.[10, 33]

There is a great financial and environmental cost to AI/ML development and use. The training of deep neural networks, today's gold standard in ML, involves vast amounts of data and electricity for computation. Training GPT-3's predecessor GPT-2 generated 315 times the amount of carbon dioxide as one passenger on a flight from New York to San Francisco.[34]

The SARS Covid-19 pandemic that gripped the world in 2020 and continues to do so at the time of writing in late 2021 presented the perfect opportunity for AI/ML to prove its real-world utility. The opportunity ranged from predicting geographical outbreaks to tools for diagnosis and prognosis.

A systematic review of 169 studies covering 232 (diagnostic and prognostic) prediction models concluded that only two met standards rigorous enough for validation across multiple cohorts.[35] The rest suffered with numerous methodological problems, including a high risk of unclear bias and model overfitting. Overfitting occurs when a ML model learns the patterns in the training data so well that it cannot generalise to new unseen data.

Another systematic review looking at ML models for the diagnosis or prognosis of Covid-19 from Chest X-ray or CT images found that none of the 62 studies meeting inclusion criteria were suitable for clinical use. This study used the Checklist for Artificial Intelligence in Medical Imaging (CLAIM),[36] which is a 42-item checklist for study reporting adapted from the Standards for Reporting of Diagnostic Accuracy Studies (STARD). Roberts et al. indicated that most studies failed to explain how they selected models, prepared images for ML or included enough detail to enable replication of the learning process itself.[37]

The rise of AI/ML has coincided with the age of privacy and data ownership. Laws around the world dictate the way in which organisations can use the data they hold of individuals. The Data Protection Act 2018 is the UK's implementation of the General Data Protection Regulation (GDPR).[38] In the United States, the Health Insurance Portability and Accountability Act of 1996 (HIPAA) is a federal law that required the creation of national standards to protect sensitive patient health information from being disclosed without the patient's consent or knowledge.[39]

The recognition that personally identifiable information has inherent value to the individual makes it a challenging subject matter for AI/ML. Data is the fuel of AI/ML, endowing it with apparent superpowers. It is no surprise that there has effectively been a gold rush for clinical data to capture the flag of healthcare AI/ML.

Big business, AI and public healthcare data have a difficult time mixing. In 2016, DeepMind made an agreement with the Royal Free London to develop an application that could detect the earliest signs of acute kidney failure. The agreement involved the sharing of 1.6 million patient records. Although assurances were given that this data would only be used for the purposes of the application, mistrust did significant reputational damage to DeepMind and Google in the healthcare space in the UK. The UK's Information Commissioner's Office would later rule that 'Royal Free NHS Foundation Trust failed to comply with the Data Protection Act when it provided patient details to Google DeepMind'.[40]

IBM has also courted controversy when in 2017 it reached an agreement with the Italian government to share clinical records of 61 million Italians.[41]

To complete a hattrick, fears over healthcare AI as implemented by Babylon Health were highlighted to the Medicines and Healthcare products Regulatory Agency (MHRA) by a consultant oncologist. The oncologist raised concerns over the 'apparent absence of any robust clinical testing or validation'. In December 2020, the MHRA would write to Dr Watkins, stating 'Your concerns are all valid and ones that we share'.[42]

The Mitigations

Using AI safely involves a combination of the acquisition and application of knowledge and experience. Knowledge comes from carefully studying how AI works and studying the mistakes that have already been made. Experience comes from a willingness to be bold, innovate and apply ML and AI in areas that would otherwise potentially get left behind.

There are a range of frameworks and principles in place to make AI and ML safe in general and in healthcare. In the UK, no single organisation has responsibility for AI regulation in healthcare. The MHRA regulates their safety, the Health Research Authority

(HRA) oversees the research to generate evidence, the National Institute for Health and Care Excellence (NICE) assesses their value, to determine whether they should be deployed, and the Care Quality Commission (CQC) must ensure that healthcare providers follow the best practice in using AI.[43] The MHRA treats clinical AI applications as AI as a medical device (AIaMD), an extension of Software as a Medical Device (SaMD).[44] Revision of how AIaMD is regulated is currently in progress.[44] This revision is necessary as the Medical Devices Regulations 2002 which governed software were not designed to regulate intelligent applications. Current regulation is linked to the function of the device and classifying the risk of harm in utilising the medical device:[45]

Class I – generally regarded as low risk

Class IIa – generally regarded as medium risk

Class IIb – generally regarded as medium risk

Class III – generally regarded as high risk.

The evidence standards framework (ESF) for digital health technologies produced by NICE treats AIaMD as digital health technologies (DHT).[46] The ESF takes an approach which classifies DHTs based on their function:

- Tier A: System services that do not directly impact patient care.
- Tier B: Applications that provide or record data or facilitate communication between 'citizens, patients or healthcare professionals'.
- Tier C: Applications that diagnose/guide diagnoses, actively monitor, calculate, facilitate self-management/behaviour change or treat/guide treatment.

Importantly, the ESF only applies to AI using fixed algorithms – algorithms that do not change once they have been trained – and excludes adaptive algorithms – algorithms capable of additional learning whilst in use.

The Standard Protocol Items: Recommendations for Interventional Trials–Artificial Intelligence (SPIRIT-AI) is an additional checklist item to address AI-specific content that is not adequately covered by SPIRIT 2013,[47] which in turn provides minimum guidance applicable for all clinical trial interventions. Nine of the 15 AI-related additions are added with respect to methodological transparency. Rather than simply stating one 'interventional group was exposed to the AI and the other was not', details such as algorithm version, data acquisition and input criteria as well as the role of humans is required.

The Consolidated Standards of Reporting Trials–Artificial Intelligence (CONSORT-AI) was developed along with SPIRIT-AI.[48] It is an extension to CONSORT, adding 14 items, and like SPIRIT-AI requiring more transparency in reporting methodology.

There are other frameworks such as CLAIM, Transparent Reporting of a multivariable prediction model for Individual Prognosis or Diagnosis (TRIPOD),[49] Prediction model Risk Of Bias Assessment Tool (PROBAST),[50] and Quality Assessment of Diagnostic Accuracy Studies (QUADAS).[51]

In moving from research to implementation, the UK government has published *A Guide to Good Practice for Digital and Data-Driven Health Technologies*.[52] This guidance helpfully highlights the areas that should be considered in delivering ML/AI tools in healthcare. Importantly, it also points out the regulatory organisations that need to be consulted and complied with (in the UK) such as the MHRA and Care Quality Commission. Most jurisdictions around the world that have worked out some regulatory frameworks for the development and deployment of AI/ML applications in healthcare have only done so in recent years.

In May 2020, the Information Commissioner's Office (ICO) published *Explaining Decisions Made with AI* in conjunction with the Alan Turing Institute.[53] This provides an in-depth understanding of how AI decisions are made for data protection officers and compliance officers, technical teams and senior management in organisations utilising AI/ML to make decisions. The guidance identifies six main types of explanation:

- **Rationale explanation**: the reasons that led to a decision, delivered in an accessible and non-technical way.
- **Responsibility explanation**: who is involved in the development, management and implementation of an AI system, and who to contact for a human review of a decision?
- **Data explanation**: what data has been used in a particular decision and how?
- **Fairness explanation**: the steps taken across the design and implementation of an AI system to ensure that the decisions it supports are generally unbiased and fair, and whether or not an individual has been treated equitably.
- **Safety and performance explanation**: the steps taken across the design and implementation of an AI system to maximise the accuracy, reliability, security and robustness of its decisions and behaviours.
- **Impact explanation**: the steps taken across the design and implementation of an AI system to consider and monitor the impacts that the use of an AI system and its decisions has or may have on an individual and on wider society.

Specific weaknesses such as bias can be addressed during the model development process using tools such as the What-If Tool (WIT),[54] IBM AI Fairness 360,[55] Local Interpretable Model-Agnostic Explanations[56] and FairML.[57] These tools allow researchers and developers to examine the variables that influence the outputs of ML algorithms and hence identify the source of bias and provide an opportunity to remove it.

Organisations that create AI services need to take responsibility for its risks. OpenAI, for example, requires that customers using its GPT-3 language model apply safety practices.[58] These include filtering sensitive and unsafe content and taking steps to keep the application on topic; it should not be used in healthcare diagnostics. This limits clinical application of GPT-3 but does not prevent the development of clinically useful language models using the same techniques. This has been done with BEHRT (BERT[59] for Electronic Health Records), a model which uses a patient's past Electronic Health Record to predict their potential future diagnoses.[60]

Another way to reduce the risks involved in AI/ML in healthcare is to collate reports on adverse incidents in and outside of healthcare.[61] The AI Incident Database describes itself as the only collection of AI deployment harms or near harms across all disciplines, geographies and use cases.[62] It facilitates the submission of such incidents by ordinary people.

What Does the Future Hold?

The future will hopefully make safe AI in psychiatry more accessible. The professionals who work in the field of AI and ML are still in demand. There have been multiple demonstrations of tools that transcribe clinical letters whilst listening to psychiatrists speak to their patients. The developments in NLP will eventually lead to naturally sounding artificial clinicians.

Rather than fearing that these will replace human clinicians, it may be possible that they would replicate individual clinicians as assistants, allowing them to attend to more patients.

Funding for digital mental health businesses reached $5.1 billion in 2021 – more than any other clinical indication and having risen from $0.5 billion in 2017.[63]

Knowledge about how to develop ML and AI tools is widely available, increasing the chance that novel ideas and solutions will come from unlikely sources. Organisations such as AI for Good[64] and the Distributed AI Research Institute[65] facilitate democratisation of specialist knowledge that would otherwise be tied up by large corporations.

Summary

The potential of AI still attracts polarising views. There are clear benefits and dangers. The key is being aware of what these are and understanding that it is possible to utilise AI in psychiatry safely. There has to be a will to do so as it is far more expensive to develop AI applications safely than it is to develop them at all. As shown, however, there are hidden costs that make this a false economy.

Ultimately, transparency about the inner workings of AI/ML tools makes increasing their safety realistic. It reduces the sense of magic but that is a small price to pay.

References

1. Fantasia. *IMDb*. 1940. Available at: www .imdb.com/title/tt0032455/?ref_=fn_al_ tt_1 (accessed 3 February 2022).

2. Artificial intelligence. *Cambridge Dictionary*. Available at: https://dictionary .cambridge.org/dictionary/english/artifi cial-intelligence (accessed 1 November 2021).

3. Machine learning. *Cambridge Dictionary*. Available at: https://dictionary.cambridge.or g/dictionary/english/machine-learning (accessed 19 November 2022).

4. Department of Health & Social Care. *Accelerating Artificial Intelligence in Health and Care: Results from a State of the Nation Survey*. 2018. Available at: https://wessexahsn.org.uk/img/news/ AHSN%20Network%20AI%20 Report-1536078823.pdf (accessed 3 February 2022).

5. Shatte, A. B. R., Hutchinson, D. M., Teague, S. J. Machine learning in mental health: a scoping review of methods and applications. *Psychol. Med.* 2019;49(9): 1426–48.

6. Rosenfeld, A., Benrimoh, D., Armstrong, C. et al. Big data analytics and AI in mental healthcare. 2019. Available at: https://arxiv.org/abs/1903.12071 (accessed 2 February 2022).

7. Jones, S. S., Heaton, P. S., Rudin, R. S., Schneider, E. C. Unraveling the IT productivity paradox: lessons for health care. *N. Engl. J. Med.* 2012;366(24): 2243–5.

8. The King's Fund. *Mental Health under Pressure*. 2015. Available at: www .kingsfund.org.uk/sites/default/files/field/ field_publication_file/mental-health-under-pressure-nov15_0.pdf (accessed 10 July 2022).

9. Abbe, A., Grouin, C., Zweigenbaum, P., Falissard, B. Text mining applications in psychiatry: a systematic literature review. *Int. J. Methods Psychiatr. Res.* 2016;25(2): 86–100.

10. GPT-3. A robot wrote this entire article. Are you scared yet, human? *The Guardian*, 8 September 2020. Available at: www .theguardian.com/commentisfree/2020/ sep/08/robot-wrote-this-article-gpt-3 (accessed 21 July 2021).

11. Smith, A. Microsoft patent shows plans to revive dead loved ones as chatbots. *Independent*, 20 January 2021. Available at: www.independent.co.uk/life-style/gadgets-

and-tech/microsoft-chatbot-patent-dead-b1789979.html (accessed 3 February 2022).

12. Fitzpatrick, K. K., Darcy, A., Vierhile, M. Delivering cognitive behavior therapy to young adults with symptoms of depression and anxiety using a fully automated conversational agent (Woebot): a randomized controlled trial. *JMIR Ment. Health.* 2017;4(2): e19.

13. Inkster, B., Sarda, S., Subramanian, V. An empathy-driven, conversational artificial intelligence agent (Wysa) for digital mental well-being: real-world data evaluation mixed-methods study. *JMIR mHealth and uHealth.* 2018;6(11): e12106.

14. Luxton, D. D. *Artificial Intelligence in Behavioral and Mental Health Care.* 1st ed. Cambridge, MA: Academic Press. 2015.

15. Mehltretter, J., Fratila, R., Benrimoh, D. A. et al. Differential treatment benefit prediction for treatment selection in depression: a deep learning analysis of STAR*D and CO-MED data. *Comput. Psychiatry.* 2020;4(0): 61.

16. Walsh, C. G., Ribeiro, J. D., Franklin, J. C. Predicting suicide attempts in adolescents with longitudinal clinical data and machine learning. *J. Child Psychol. Psychiatry.* 2018;59(12): 1261–70.

17. Rumshisky, A., Ghassemi, M., Naumann, T. et al. Predicting early psychiatric readmission with natural language processing of narrative discharge summaries. *Transl. Psychiatry.* 2016;6(10): e921.

18. Banoula, M. Bias and variance in machine learning: an in depth explanation. *Simplilearn.* 2021. Available at: www .simplilearn.com/tutorials/machine-learning-tutorial/bias-and-variance (accessed 25 September 2021).

19. Jones, T. Machine learning and bias. *IBM Developer.* 2019. Available at: https:// developer.ibm.com/articles/machine-learning-and-bias/ (accessed 25 September 2021).

20. Obermeyer, Z., Powers, B., Vogeli, C., Mullainathan, S. Dissecting racial bias in an algorithm used to manage the health of populations. *Science.* 2019;366(6464): 447–53.

21. Gov.UK. Detentions under the Mental Health Act. 2021. Available at: www .ethnicity-facts-figures.service.gov.uk/ health/mental-health/detentions-under-the-mental-health-act/latest (accessed 3 February 2022).

22. Olbert, C. M., Nagendra, A., Buck, B. Meta-analysis of Black vs. White racial disparity in schizophrenia diagnosis in the United States: do structured assessments attenuate racial disparities? *J. Abnorm. Psychol.* 2018;127(1): 104–15.

23. Sansone, R. A., Sansone, L. A. Gender patterns in borderline personality disorder. *Innov. Clin. Neurosci.* 2011;8(5): 16–20.

24. Dalgleish, T., Power, M. *Handbook of Cognition and Emotion.* 1st ed. Chichester: Wiley. 2007.

25. Chen, L., Ma, X., Zhu, N. et al. Facial expression recognition with machine learning and assessment of distress in patients with cancer. *Oncol. Nurs. Forum.* 2021;48(1): 81–93.

26. Buolamwini, J., Gebru, T. Gender shades: intersectional accuracy disparities in commercial gender classification. In Sorelle, A., Friedler, C. W., eds, *Proceedings of the 1st Conference on Fairness, Accountability and Transparency.* New York: Proceedings of Machine Learning Research. 2018. pp. 77–91.

27. BBC News. IBM abandons 'biased' facial recognition tech. 9 June 2020. Available at: www.bbc.co.uk/news/technology-5297819 1 (accessed 23 November 2021).

28. Murgia, M. Microsoft quietly deletes largest public face recognition data set. *Financial Times,* 6 June 2019. Available at: www.ft.com/content/7d3e0d6a-87a0-11e9-a028-86cea8523dc2 (accessed 23 November 2022).

29. Jin, B., Qu, Y., Zhang, L., Gao, Z. Diagnosing Parkinson disease through facial expression recognition: video analysis. *J. Med. Internet Res.* 2020;22(7): e18697.

30. Orme, J. Samaritans pulls 'suicide watch' Radar app over privacy concerns. *The*

Guardian, 7 November 2014. Available at: www.theguardian.com/society/2014/nov/07/samaritans-radar-app-suicide-watch-privacy-twitter-users (accessed 14 July 2021).

31. Lee, D. Tay: Microsoft issues apology over racist chatbot fiasco. *BBC News*, 25 March 2016. Available at: www.bbc.co.uk/news/technology-35902104 (accessed 5 February 2022).

32. Mellor, D. What are the emerging risks of AI? *Swiss Re*, 3 December 2020. Available at: https://corporatesolutions.swissre.com/insights/knowledge/emerging-risks-of-AI.html (accessed 3 February 2022).

33. Cahn, A. F. A human wrote this article. You shouldn't be scared of GPT-3. *The Guardian*, 12 September 2020. Available at: www.theguardian.com/commentisfree/2020/sep/12/human-wrote-this-article-gpt-3 (accessed 21 July 2021).

34. Strubell, E., Ganesh, A., McCallum, A. Energy and policy considerations for deep learning in NLP. 2019 Jun 5 arXiv preprint arXiv:1906.02243.

35. Wynants, L., van Calster, B., Collins, G. S. et al. Prediction models for diagnosis and prognosis of Covid-19: systematic review and critical appraisal. *BMJ*. 2020;7: m1328.

36. Mongan, J., Moy, L., Kahn, C. E. Checklist for Artificial Intelligence in Medical Imaging (CLAIM): a guide for authors and reviewers. *Radiol. Artif. Intell.* 2020;2(2): e200029.

37. Roberts, M., Driggs, D., Thorpe, M. et al. Common pitfalls and recommendations for using machine learning to detect and prognosticate for COVID-19 using chest radiographs and CT scans. *Nat. Mach. Intell.* 2021;3(3): 199–217.

38. ICO. *Guide to the UK General Data Protection Regulation (UK GDPR)*. n.d. Available at: https://ico.org.uk/for-organisations/guide-to-data-protection/guide-to-the-general-data-protection-regulation-gdpr/ (accessed 10 July 2021).

39. Health Insurance Portability and Accountability Act of 1996 (HIPAA). *CDC*. Available at: www.cdc.gov/phlp/publica

tions/topic/hipaa.html (accessed 3 February 2022).

40. ICO. The Information Commissioner's Office response to the Department for Digital, Culture, Media and Sport's consultation on the National Data Strategy. n.d. Available at: https://ico.org.uk/media/about-the-ico/consultation-responses/2618963/ico-response-national-data-strategy-consultation.pdf (accessed 3 February 2022).

41. Moody, G. Detailed medical records of 61 million Italian citizens to be given to IBM for its 'cognitive computing' system Watson. *LaptrinhX*, 23 May 2017. Available at: https://laptrinhx.com/detailed-medical-records-of-61-million-italian-citizens-to-be-given-to-ibm-for-its-cognitive-computing-system-watson-3962904859/ (accessed 3 February 2022).

42. Carding, N. Regulator reveals 'concerns' over Babylon's 'chatbot'. *HSJ*. 2021. Available at: www.hsj.co.uk/technology-and-innovation/regulator-reveals-concerns-over-babylons-chatbot/7029598.article? (accessed 3 February 2023).

43. Iacobucci, G. Row over Babylon's chatbot shows lack of regulation. *BMJ*. 2020;368: m815.

44. Medicines and Healthcare products Regulatory Agency. *Software and AI as a Medical Device Change Programme*. 2021. Available at: www.gov.uk/government/publications/software-and-ai-as-a-medical-device-change-programme/software-and-ai-as-a-medical-device-change-programme (accessed 3 February 2022).

45. Grainger, D. Guidance: Medical device stand-alone software including apps (including IVDMDs) v1.08. Available at: https://assets.publishing.service.gov.uk/government/uploads/system/uploads/attachment_data/file/999908/Software_flow_chart_Ed_1-08b-IVD.pdf (accessed 3 February 2022).

46. National Institute for Health and Care Excellence (NICE). Evidence standards framework for digital health technologies. Available at: www.nice.org.uk/about/what-we-do/our-programmes/evidence-

standards-framework-for-digital-health-technologies (accessed 17 March 2022).

47. Cruz Rivera, S., Liu, X., Chan, A-W. et al. Guidelines for clinical trial protocols for interventions involving artificial intelligence: the SPIRIT-AI extension. *Lancet Digit. Health.* 2020;2(10): e549–60.

48. Liu, X., Rivera, S. C., Moher, D., Calvert, M. J., Denniston, A. K. Reporting guidelines for clinical trial reports for interventions involving artificial intelligence: the CONSORT-AI Extension. *BMJ.* 2020;370: m3164.

49. Collins, G. S., Reitsma, J. B., Altman, D. G., Moons, K. G. M. Transparent Reporting of a multivariable prediction model for Individual Prognosis Or Diagnosis (TRIPOD): the TRIPOD statement. *Br. J. Surg.* 2015;102(3): 148–58.

50. Moons, K. G. M., Wolff, R. F., Riley, R. D. et al. PROBAST: a tool to assess risk of bias and applicability of prediction model studies: explanation and elaboration. *Ann. Intern. Med.* 2019;170(1): W1.

51. Whiting, P. F. QUADAS-2: a revised tool for the quality assessment of diagnostic accuracy studies. *Ann. Intern. Med.* 2011;155(8): 529.

52. Department of Health & Social Care. *A Guide to Good Practice for Digital and Data-Driven Health Technologies.* 2021. Available at: www.gov.uk/government/publications/code-of-conduct-for-data-driven-health-and-care-technology/initial-code-of-conduct-for-data-driven-health-and-care-technology (accessed 3 February 2022).

53. ICO. Explaining decisions made with AI. n. d. Available at: https://ico.org.uk/for-organisations/guide-to-data-protection/key-dp-themes/explaining-decisions-made-with-artificial-intelligence/ (accessed 3 February 2022).

54. PAIR-code/what-if-tool: source code/webpage/demos for the What-If Tool. Available at: https://github.com/pair-code/what-if-tool (accessed 3 February 2022).

55. Trusted-AI/AIF360: a comprehensive set of fairness metrics for datasets and machine learning models, explanations for these metrics, and algorithms to mitigate bias in datasets and models. Available at: https://github.com/Trusted-AI/AIF360 (accessed 3 February 2022).

56. marcotcr/lime: Lime: explaining the predictions of any machine learning classifier. Available at: https://github.com/marcotcr/lime (accessed 3 February 2022).

57. adebayoj/fairml. Available at: https://github.com/adebayoj/fairml (accessed 3 February 2022).

58. OpenAI. Safety best practices – OpenAI API. n.d. Available at: https://beta.openai.com/docs/safety-best-practices (accessed 21 July 2021).

59. Devlin, J., Chang, M-W., Lee, K., Toutanova, K. BERT: pre-training of deep bidirectional transformers for language understanding. arXiv preprint arXiv:1810.04805.

60. Li, Y., Rao, S., Solares, J. R. A. et al. BEHRT: transformer for electronic health records. *Sci. Rep.* 2020;10(1): 7155.

61. Challen, R., Denny, J., Pitt, M., Gompels, L., Edwards, T., Tsaneva-Atanasova, K. Artificial intelligence, bias and clinical safety. *BMJ Qual. Saf.* 2019;28 (3): 231–7.

62. AI Incident Database. Welcome to the Artificial Intelligence Incident Database. n. d. Available at: https://incidentdatabase.ai/?lang=en (accessed 3 February 2022).

63. Rock Health. 2021 year-end digital health funding: seismic shifts beneath the surface. 10 January 2022. Available at: https://rockhealth.com/insights/2021-year-end-digital-health-funding-seismic-shifts-beneath-the-surface/ (accessed 3 February 2022).

64. AI for Good. n.d. Available at: www.aiforgood.co.uk/about-us (accessed 3 February 2022).

65. The DAIR Institute. Available at: www.dair-institute.org/ (accessed 3 February 2022).

Chapter 6

Digital Clinicians
Growing a Different Type of Healthcare Professional

James Reed and Omer Moghraby

In regione caecorum rex est luscus.
Credited to Desiderius Erasmus's Adagia,[1] *1500*

In the country of the blind, the one-eyed man is king.
Anon

Introduction

The quote above describes the experience of most mental health clinicians who have found themselves working in what are still variously described and ill-defined roles in a field which also struggles to define itself. Various names have surfaced – 'clinical informatics' and 'digital health' being the most popular, and to match a dizzying array of job roles and titles – 'clinical director for informatics', 'clinical lead for technology', 'clinical informatician' and so on.

The relatively slow pace of change in the way that medicine is practised in secondary care has meant that it is only now that the need for 'expert users' who understand both the clinical work and the systems that are intended to support it has been recognised. As clinical systems and technology move from novelties into core tools, so it is now time for psychiatrists interested in this area to move from enthusiastic amateurs into trained professionals.

It is also clear that all mental health clinicians, whatever their interest in systems and technology, will now be expected to use these tools in their daily work and are likely to need to develop their own skills to make best use of them. Just as we have adjusted over decades of practice to new technology (most notably the introduction of effective medication from the 1950s), it is now time for another significant shift in the way we do our work.

We will cover recent history and trace the development of the clinical leader through to the emergence of the role of 'Chief Clinical Information Officer' (commonly abbreviated to 'CCIO') and beyond. We will explore how this can be developed further and how training should be expanded both at the beginning of medical careers and through to senior roles. We will consider what new skills will be needed by all clinical staff and how these can be nurtured and developed, and we will look ahead to what the practice of psychiatry will be like in the coming years.

Recent History: From Zero to Hero

As recently as the early 2010s, it was still rare to find practising clinicians also working on developing and improving the use of technology in their work. Such ideas were regarded by many as something of an eccentricity, and people working in it regarded with an indulgent eye and known as 'being good with computers'. Those attempting to pursue this interest rapidly became familiar with colleagues asking for advice on subjects ranging from why their keyboard or mouse isn't working through to weightier matters such as the shortcomings of the spell checker in Microsoft Word.

In general practice, these clinicians were able to relatively easily introduce changes to their practices because of the small scale and the fact they were sometimes the owners of the business. All of the main GP systems currently in existence grew out of the work of pioneering GPs who coded the clinical systems themselves (notably Dr David Stables and Dr Peter Sowerby, the co-founders of EMIS). However, clinicians working in secondary care with similar skills did not have the same level of opportunity and control to bring changes and 'computerisation' consisted of large mainframe computers which processed administrative data. Some hospitals made strides – for example, Reaside Clinic in Birmingham specified and installed a full-scale Electronic Health Record in the early 1990s on the basis that the (then emerging) new specialty of 'forensic psychiatry' needed legible notes.

The desire to bring a similar level of digital maturity to secondary care led to the ill-fated National Programme for IT (NPfIT), which is discussed in detail in Chapter 1. One of the reasons for its failure was the lack of clinical leadership and engagement.[2] A small number of heroic figures did everything possible to avert disaster, but in retrospect it is clear that the emphasis was placed far too much on big technology companies and the role for clinical experts in design and implementation was overlooked. Mental health providers did better than others in this regard and working systems were delivered. Some pioneering mental health clinicians found themselves in leadership roles, but this was not recognised at a regional or national level.

However, at grassroots level there were some signs of change. A small but vocal website which was known as a prominent critic of the NPfIT ('e-health insider[*]') began to socialise the concept commonly seen in the United States of a 'Chief Medical Information Officer', a senior clinician (at that time usually a doctor) with responsibility for overseeing the design and operation of electronic records systems. The term 'Chief Clinical Information Officer' was coined, and a campaign established to lobby for every NHS provider organisation to appoint a CCIO to provide clinical leadership on suggest 'technology' instead - IM&T is jargon and unless defined elsewhere in th book might not be clear projects. From the outset the idea was to broaden the scope from being purely a medical role to being one that anyone with a clinical background could fulfil.

This campaign proved to be very successful and captured a new wave of enthusiasm as people began to turn from looking back at failures to looking ahead to what might be done next. The promise was to bring clinical leadership to the fore. The campaign evolved into more formal networks, supported by conferences and online discussion forums. Mental health organisations were frequently seen to be leading the way and many prominent figures within the networks were from this field.

The role of CCIO has become increasingly well established, and whilst by no means every organisation has such an appointment it is now increasingly rare to find NHS trusts

---

[*] www.ehi.co.uk/ (now defunct)

without some form of clinical leadership of systems and technology. However, the current cadre are largely those who have spent considerable time in this area as it has developed, and career paths remain somewhat unclear, as does the route for development for those earlier in their careers.

Training and Development

Undergraduate

The rapid growth of technology in clinical practice has not been matched by developments in undergraduate curricula. Medical schools and related higher education establishments generally do not list specific informatics modules or competencies as part of their course structures and there is no consensus on what undergraduates should be taught. The experience of technology in clinical placements will vary widely, and any teaching there is likely to be based around particular products or local processes rather than principles.

It will be necessary to walk a tightrope between practicalities (which may be biased too far towards particular systems or products) and principles (which may be too theoretical to be useful). There are also questions to be addressed about selecting medical students – given that they are entering an increasingly technical profession, should aptitude and skills be assessed at that stage?

The same questions need to be considered when constructing undergraduate placements. There has been much debate about improving recruitment through providing an inspiring experience but it is also important to ensure that students receive positive messages about all aspects of practice. Mental health services are frequently more digitally mature than acute hospitals, and it would be unfortunate if they come away from placements with a negative view of it. In addition, there are often considerable difficulties in arranging access for students to clinical systems, given that they are not usually considered as employees, the placements are short and system training is usually needed before accounts can be set up. Little attention is paid to the clinical design of systems or how they can best be used to support care. Instead, they are largely considered of no greater status than a file of notes would have been in traditional education.

Much has been made in popular culture of the difference between 'digital immigrants' (those who grew up before the advent of the 'digital age' and who have had to learn new skills) and 'digital natives' – those who have grown up with technology and know no different. It is not clear that this logic has followed through for 'digital natives' to naturally adopt systems in their work and be keen to develop them further. The definition is constantly shifting (e.g. from children of the 1970s who grew up with microcomputers, to children of the early 2000s who have grown up with the World Wide Web or even to children of the 2010s who have grown up with social media). This is also true of any assumptions that younger generations are more interested or skilled with technology than older generations. The definitions of what is regarded as technology, especially in current healthcare, is also shifting. Technology as a commodity may further alienate those whom we may assume would be best place to use it.

Learning within the context of medical schools or healthcare (especially professional) education needs to evolve with these changes and include aspects of care that will be delivered with the support of, or through, technology (however that is defined). It is relevant for students to start to develop the skills to understand its utility, evaluate the delivery of outcomes and also ways to innovate practice to improve healthcare.

Universities should be at the forefront of innovative teaching methods, particularly in terms of simulating clinical encounters. There are great opportunities here although as yet they do not appear to have been exploited fully, if at all.

Postgraduate

Turning to postgraduate, there are similar questions to address. For psychiatrists, the core psychiatry RCPsych curriculum makes minimal mention of the issue;[3] the 2019 curriculum listed only a single skill in one domain referring to 'use appropriate IT skills' without any further explanation. The 2022 curriculum removes even that, replacing it with vague references to 'new technology' (which in itself seems difficult to apply to electronic patient records). There are also mentions made of record keeping and documentation, but these are again limited and without detail. Whilst trainees will undoubtedly be exposed to clinical systems in their organisations, there is no definition of what skills are needed or how these can be developed. Specifically, the paradigm remains that of paper records and as yet psychiatric training does not address the transformative angle to employing technology.

There are similar issues in higher training curricula at present. There is a clear opportunity for specialty areas to develop specific skills which will be relevant. For example, forensic psychiatry could address the specific security angles of consumer technology in secure hospitals, or general adult or child psychiatry might include competencies in conducting assessments over video calls, or how to evaluate engagement.

There may even be scope for entirely new subspeciality areas. 'Digital clinicians' might be practitioners who develop particular skills in remote assessment and the use of other supportive technologies (video calls/text messages/computer-based therapies etc). However, this approach might also run the risk of these skills being insufficiently developed in the traditional specialty areas.

Alongside developing new ways of working clinically, there is also a need for access to experience and training in providing clinical leadership to development of clinical systems. This might be done through special interest sessions with established local clinical leadership to enable practice through project work. There have also been a number of training courses (short and long) developed to supplement this training or facilitate more formal learning – either as a part of training or in addition to it (not unlike traditional therapeutic training, e.g. systemic and family therapy training). Over recent years, there has been a determined effort to establish other career pathways (such as fellowships in academic medicine or medical education) with well-funded training programmes often associated with formal qualifications such as higher degrees. These have allowed those with an interest to develop their skills in a manner which is well-recognised and allows parallel development with clinical work.

A similar 'digital clinician' pathway might be developed in conjunction with universities and industry, but this will require interest from current leaders in the profession and considerable investment to bring to fruition.

Senior Positions

Such has been the pace of development over recent years that most doctors working in this area have few if any formal qualifications in health informatics or related subjects. Such qualifications that do exist (e.g. MSc courses) tend to be more focused on data science than leadership and management of technology within a healthcare organisation. The reality of working in these posts is that these skills are little used – instead the focus is on change management, human factors and deep understanding of systems and organisations. The stereotype of the CCIO is someone 'good with computers', but a far more important and relevant skill is that of being 'good with people'. Most working in CCIO or equivalent posts have come into them by chance and usually in response to a sudden need (such as the implementation of a new health information system, e.g. ePMA). The general level of digital maturity within mental health trusts is improving, and therefore this particular route is unlikely to remain available in the long run.

The most common career pathway for UK psychiatrists is through basic and higher specialist training, culminating in a consultant post with similar pathways to manager or consultant for other professional groups. Thereafter it becomes less well defined, but many develop recognised and funded interests in research, medical education, management and other areas. For those aspiring to develop as digital leaders, the pathways are not clear and even the posts may vary from one organisation to another. Not all organisations have formal posts in this area, and for those that do the status of the posts, the renumeration and the amount of time allocated are widely variable.

This poses two problems – the first is that there is no clear pathway for clinicians who want to work in digital health to follow. The increasingly structured nature of training requires clinicians to pick a subspecialty at a relatively early stage, and whilst there are sometimes 'special interests' available, this is not likely to be reliable or consistent across the country. There is hence a high risk that keen clinicians become frustrated and lose interest, and they may rightly be concerned that spending time attempting to pursue such a career is disadvantaging them.

The second is that those currently in post as CCIOs are unlikely to be satisfied with remaining in the same post for a long period of time. Whilst this will vary according to the individual, anyone wishing to further their career will need to have a pathway to aspire towards. At present, CCIOs usually report directly to an executive director. Therefore, the next obvious step would be for these roles to be in an executive position. The experience gained as a CCIO, as they are currently configured, is unlikely to provide sufficient operational management exposure to lead to a successful appointment as, for instance, an executive medical director. Without obvious succession planning or pathways for individuals, it has led to departures from involvement in digital health leadership. There is therefore a risk of a 'brain drain' out of digital health.

Some CCIO posts have equivalent status to clinical directors or deputy medical directors with multiple dedicated sessions and generous responsibility allowances. Others may have no dedicated time, sit outside the regular management structure and attract little or no additional payments. The latter require a considerable amount of goodwill and also senior support if they are to have any impact. Whilst there have been efforts made by central NHS bodies to endorse the concept of clinical leadership posts in systems and technology, there is no requirement for providers to have such posts. The main catalyst for investment in such posts is usually a large implementation project, typically for a new electronic patient record system, and many of the larger system suppliers expect such posts to be in place when embarking on such projects.

Some executive medical director posts also carry the badge of CCIO but these are largely regarded as a ceremonial appointments as (albeit with some exceptions) it is extremely difficult for medical directors to devote sufficient time and attention to digital health leadership. A similar phenomenon has been seen when the NHS regional medical directors in England were given the title of CCIO without any clarity on what this meant. Perhaps unsurprisingly this move has led to little actual change, and those organisations who have added digital health to the medical director's portfolio without additional resourcing have seen little progress being made.

The NHS Long Term Plan noted as a milestone that in 2021/22 there would be a CIO or CCIO on the board, but as yet there has been little evidence of this. A very small number of individuals have gained executive posts as 'Chief Digital Information Officers' although these are the exception, and it remains to be seen if there will be further such appointments.

NHS Digital Academy

The need for equipping those currently working in digital health with knowledge and skills whilst at the same time offering a solid grounding for those aspiring to such careers was recognised in the formation of the NHS Digital Academy in the UK. This followed directly from a recommendation in the Wachter Report,[4] which was described in Chapter 1. It recommended that the workforce be provided with support and training, and specifically that there should be efforts to 'create and certify training programmes for clinician-informaticians'.

The Academy was conceived as an equivalent to other training programmes within the public sector with specific aims (e.g. the 'Major Projects Leadership Academy'). It was established with academic partners at Imperial College London (initially also in conjunction with Edinburgh University and Harvard University) and set out to deliver a programme of training culminating in a formal qualification (a postgraduate diploma or Master's degree). The Academy was founded in 2017 with the first cohort starting in 2018 and the programme has been running annually since. The programme covers a range of areas including generic topics (leadership, project management) and those more specific to digital health (data analytics, user-centred design, etc.). The response to the programme from those who have completed it has been generally positive, although one of the main criticisms of the programme as a whole is that the number of places available remains small (around 100 per cohort) and the applications process is highly competitive, making it difficult to secure a place.

The main programme is likely to continue to run although there is also likely to be a wider range of training offered under the 'Digital Academy' branding. The devolved nations are looking at similar approaches, either buying places on the NHS England Digital Academy or setting up their own as Scotland has in 2023.

Topol Fellowships

The Topol Fellowships have developed in parallel to the Digital Academy although ostensibly the aims are similar. They had their origin in another review by another US physician (Dr Eric Topol), who was invited by a different Secretary of State for Health although the focus of the review was on what was needed to develop the workforce with appropriate skills in digital heath. The practical outworking of this was the establishment of year-long fellowships, in which a relatively small cohort of individuals (approximately 35 per group) are provided with funding and protected time to deliver digital projects supported by learning and mutual support. These fellowships have also been generally well received but again the absolute numbers who benefit are small as a fraction of the workforce as a whole.

Professionalisation

Clinicians early in their careers and who wish to develop an interest in digital health may find it very difficult to know how to proceed, and to what positions they might aspire. Whilst some individuals refer to themselves as 'clinical informaticians' or similar, there is no formal specialty with that name.

However, there is now a growing recognition of the need to establish competencies and structures to allow those interested in this area to develop their career. The 'Faculty of Clinical Informatics' was established in 2015 with the intention of being 'the multi-disciplinary professional body for all health and social care qualified individuals working as informaticians across the UK'.[†] The Faculty runs events and has worked on producing various resources including a competency framework and sample job descriptions. The impact of these remains to be seen, and there is certainly no requirement to be associated with the Faculty to work in digital health at present.

However, the resources provided are likely to be of assistance both to specialist registrars wishing to develop competencies during their training and to established consultants who want to incorporate such activities into their regular work. Both those overseeing training and those acting as appraisers and responsible officers may be uncertain about how such work is recognised.

Joining the Faculty at present is based simply around an application form, and there are no formal examinations or qualification required. However, you do have to be a member of an accredited body that does have these such as the Royal Colleges. There are, however, some models in the United States which may be of relevance. The Association of Medical Directors of Informatics Systems (AMDIS) is a professional organisation specifically aimed at 'physicians interested in and responsible for health information technology' and hosts events and education materials.[‡] The College for Health Information Management Executives (CHIME) offers similar services more broadly to both health and IT professionals working in this area and offers a formal certification programme ('CHCIO').[§] CHIME is developing a presence in the UK, but this remains in its early stages and relatively few clinicians have achieved this certification.

Organisations such as the Federation for Informatics Professions (FEDIP) are working to establish core competencies across far wider groups beyond clinicians such as IT professionals working in healthcare.[**]

Career Pathways

As described above, there are clear difficulties in establishing a career pathway within existing NHS structures, and this may lead to clinicians considering other avenues for progressing. These will inevitably require them looking outside traditional NHS providers, and towards other NHS bodies or outside the NHS altogether. Historically there were several central NHS bodies in which clinicians might work including NHS Digital, NHSX and NHS England itself. In late 2021, it was announced that the first two of these would be

[†] https://facultyofclinicalinformatics.org.uk/ [‡] https://amdis.org/ [§] https://chimecentral.org/
[**] www.fedip.org/

absorbed by the third and that first two 'brands would be retired' with 'a significant reduction in workforce' - the impact is no longer unknown!. There remain a significant number of individuals with clinical backgrounds working in the centre, usually part time with substantive clinical roles. The posts involve assisting in policy development, strategy and planning. These roles provide an opportunity to have influence at high levels within the NHS management hierarchy, although they are also seen to be remote from the frontline and the impact on the delivery of clinical services can be difficult to assess.

An entirely different angle involves working in the software and technology industry. Whilst many clinicians already work in this industry, the most common pathway is for people early in their careers to leave clinical practice and either found 'startup' companies or join existing ones. These individuals gain considerable experience in technical work, but they lack expertise in any area of clinical practice and also do not have the practical experience of implementing systems within healthcare organisations. In the UK it remains unusual for technology companies to employ experienced clinicians in senior roles and as a result they often fail to appreciate many aspects of how their products are actually used, nor of the challenges that might result during or following implementation.

This need is better recognised in the United States and large companies which provide clinical software invariably employ 'physician executives' or 'chief medical officers', usually part of wider clinical teams, to advise on product design and development and to engage with customers to ensure that the products are used to their fullest extent. There is a clear need for similar developments in the UK technology industry, and in future it should be possible for experienced CCIOs to move between industry and the NHS in both directions. Unfortunately, making such a move is still regarded as risky and possibly harmful to a doctor's career, in much the same way as jobs in the pharmaceutical industry were (and in some cases still are) viewed.

There is at present an unparalleled interest in 'mental health' in society at large, and this has inspired considerable interest amongst 'startup' businesses in building products in this sector, often with the intention of selling to the NHS. They invariably have good intentions and perceive great business opportunities. Unfortunately, their lack of experience of the reality of mental health services and the NHS can lead to them becoming disillusioned and potential innovations being lost. There are opportunities for experienced CCIOs to act as advisors to these companies and assist them in in navigating the structures, as well as developing ideas for products which are likely to be genuinely useful. This is also likely to be a growth area in future but as above will rely on those with experience being willing to work in these roles, which at least in the early stages of companies' growth are unlikely to be remunerated very well or indeed at all.

Current and Future Challenges

There has been a dramatic change in the involvement of clinical staff of all backgrounds in digital leadership and as described above this has been driven by a wave of large-scale change and implementation projects. It is always much easier to find resources for this type of staffing when large projects are planned or underway (akin to 'planning for the war'). However, once the excitement has died down, the projects are completed and the organisations are facing different challenges, it can be much more difficult to justify continuing resourcing digital projects in an ongoing way. It remains important for organisations to set up a sustainable model in which staff are established in long-term posts, agnostic to any specific project delivery, with a clear strategy to deliver.

Staff engagement in general can recede. When a new system is coming in, everyone in the organisation is likely to have an opinion (positive or negative) and it is relatively straightforward to get comments, feedback and willing volunteers. As time goes on, the 'new system' become the norm and staff can lose interest. It is therefore necessary to 'plan for the peace' and develop approaches that drive continuous development and improvement.

It is becoming ever clearer that to accomplish this in any large organisation needs more than a single leader, and that what is needed is teams of 'digital clinicians' working across disciplines and services. The idea of an 'office of the CCIO', which borrows from similar concepts in the United States, is gaining traction in some quarters. The concept is that of a broad multidisciplinary team with members from both clinical and technical backgrounds who are able to lead on all aspects, with the emphasis on designing comprehensive solutions to identified clinical problems. Such an 'office' might include clinical staff from various backgrounds (doctors, nurses, psychologists, occupational therapists, etc.) working along-side software developers, business analysts, user interface designers, and so on. Such an approach is still a long journey from the way most organisations are configured and it requires vision from organisations to invest at a time when resources remain under pressure. There can be a temptation for boards to consider the work is done when the project is finished, rather than it simply being (to paraphrase Churchill) 'the end of the beginning'.

There is a significant threat that the current cadre of leaders who have experienced the excitement of the rapid phase of development over recent years may become dissatisfied if they are unable to progress further and might seek other opportunities – either by returning to mainstream medical management or seeking alternative careers in the software or consulting industries. This could in turn reduce opportunities for passing on their experience to newer staff and at worst could lead to a loss of knowledge and understanding. It is of great important that the opportunity to deliver on the immense promise afforded by 'the digital dream' is fully realised. This can only be done by investing in training at all levels and building attractive career pathways which can be followed to the most senior level.

References

1. Erasmus, D. *Erasmi Roterodami Adagiorum Chiliades Tres.* Venice. 1508. Digital Edition.

2. Justina, T. The UK's National Programme for IT: why was it dismantled? *Health Serv. Manage. Res.* 2017;30(1):2–9.

3. Royal College of Psychiatrists. Curricula and guidance. 2023. Available at: www.rcpsych.ac.uk/training/curricula-and-guidance (accessed 11 June 2023).

4. Wachter, R. M. *Making IT Work: Harnessing the Power of Health Information: Technology to Improve Care in England. Report of the National Advisory Group on Health Information Technology in England.* Department of Health. 2016. Available at: www.gov.uk/government/publications/using-information-technology-to-improve-the-nhs (accessed 19 June 2023).

Global Telepsychiatry
The Changing Face of Psychiatric Practice

Peter Yellowlees

This is an exciting and challenging time to be working in mental healthcare. Future generations of psychiatrists will provide better more accountable care and will work in a world where video is data and augmented reality is reality.

Peter Yellowlees and Jay Shore, 2018[1]

The Pre-Covid-19 Telepsychiatry World

In most countries prior to Covid-19, the suite of digital technologies from videoconferencing to mobile to apps was already transforming the practice of psychiatry.[1] This was at a slower pace than seen in other industries, such as media, banking and retail that were at the leading edge of the overall digital transformation of society, and the pace of change varied widely across countries, as it still does. Medicine and psychiatry, rather than surging into the information age, were caught at the peak of industrial age medicine, with technologies largely used to reinforce the existing systems of care rather than being implemented to change and improve them.[1] An example is the use of most Electronic Health Record (EHR) systems, which were originally built to enhance billing and administrative requirements rather than for clinical purposes, and which not surprisingly, as an unintended consequence, increased provider burnout and decreased the time available for doctor–patient interactions because of their relative lack of focus on the doctor–patient interface.

Psychiatry, globally, has gone through several waves of technology adoption.[2] The concept of distance medicine includes the use of smoke signals in medieval Europe to warn of quarantines during the Black Plague, the use of letters sent via stagecoach in the United States leading to the use of the telegraph to order medical supplies during the American Civil War, and then on to early balloons and aircraft transporting medical messages. Live interactive video conferencing, commonly referred to as telepsychiatry, began with successful demonstration projects in the United States in the early 1960s at the University of Nebraska, as well as at Massachusetts General Hospital where group therapy by video was introduced, and then on to testing mobile satellite systems developed by NASA on Indian Health reservations which were ultimately intended to assist astronauts.

This demonstration phase continued until the 1990s when a new era was spurred by revolutions in computing and the Internet around the world which significantly decreased the costs of videoconferencing, leading to potentially economically sustainable telepsychiatry services. The advent of web-based videoconferencing and the development of mobile devices and smartphones from 2007 onwards led to widespread but sporadic adoption whilst the integration of smartphone-based synchronous and asynchronous apps, EHRs and a range of virtual reality therapies have increasingly been used in conjunction with telepsychiatry.[3, 4]

Telepsychiatry has been an evidence-based practice for many years with over two decades of research and clinical guideline development supporting its use and effectiveness when compared with in-person treatments across diagnoses, settings and populations.[5-7] Two professional associations have had a specific interest in international telemedicine and telepsychiatry with long histories of collaboration and education. These are the American Telemedicine Association[8] and the International Society for Telemedicine and eHealth (ISFTeH).[9] The latter's primary focus has been in the international sector and the ISFTeH has 107 international members and partners listed on its website.

In the past decade, new models of hybrid psychiatric care have been created by blending videoconferencing across various components of health systems, including in-person care, with other technologies such as EHRs and mobile health apps using multiple passive data-collecting tools on smartphones. This has led to new virtual models of integrated care and the development of asynchronous psychiatry consultations using both EHRs and recorded patient videos. Increasingly in the United States from 2015 onwards, psychiatrists have been engaged in 'hybrid-doctor patient relationships',[3] which, post Covid-19, are increasingly common.[10]

Prior to Covid-19, there were two major global drivers of change leading to greater use of telepsychiatry and other technologies at the doctor–patient interface. These were the global move to mobile wireless devices and the impact of younger generations of patients and physicians, both of which were affecting already pronounced digital disparities across cultures and countries around the world.

Mobile devices

Since 2015, the typical smartphone has been equipped with forward-facing and rear-facing high-resolution video cameras, a high-resolution display, internet connectivity, audio inputs and outputs – via a microphone, speaker, headset port and Bluetooth connections – and advanced processing power, as well as an increasingly wide range of active and passive data collection capabilities through sensors and accelerometers. All of these features make smartphones ideal for a new class of applications providing on-the-go mobile telemental health and have changed the way that mental health services are now being delivered in most countries of the world.[11, 12]

The international trends on the use of mobile devices have been described in detail[13] and demonstrate how the mobile device, typically a smartphone, has become the new tool for the delivery of mental health services in many countries around the world. Whilst many mental health professionals in Western countries likely still use fixed computers, younger generations of physicians and mental health clinicians are rapidly switching to fully mobile devices, and in many countries these are all that is available, giving those countries, such as India and Africa, potential advantages in not having to set up and maintain wired infrastructures.[14] The global figures, as described by Deyan,[13] are astonishing and explain why such devices are the future of mental health in cyberspace and around the world.

Deyan has calculated that worldwide in 2020 there were 3.5 billion smartphone users, with 1.5 billion new smartphone sales per year, and 7.9 billion mobile broadband subscriptions (104% of the world's population) with almost 10 billion smartphones in use.[13] He noted that 67% of all internet users globally access the Internet by smartphone, whilst in the United

States 81% of citizens own smartphones and 47% say they could not live without them. In China (the leader in smartphone traffic), he reported that 99% of internet users go online using mobile devices whilst globally 56% of all website traffic in 2019 was generated by smartphones, with this projected to be 80% of global connections by smartphones by 2025.

Novel forms of interventions are more accessible than ever before anywhere in the world using smartphones. There is an extensive literature that discusses internet therapeutic interventions, including improving cognition with video games, the use of virtual reality equipment for the treatment of anxiety disorders and PTSD and internet-based cognitive therapies.[4] The common theme with these applications is the digitisation and automation of much of the range of traditional therapies, making them available to patients in between sessions with the therapist, or perhaps being supplemented by an 'avatar therapist' between sessions. Good examples built by Veterans Affairs in the United States that are freely available from the 'App store' and already widely used that act like a 'therapist in the pocket' are CBT-I Coach and PTSD Coach.[15] There is also the potential for the human therapist to be replaced entirely with a technology-based avatar that is trained to respond therapeutically to movements and language.[16]

Inter-generational Changes

The healthcare industry has been slow in adapting to the social and technological changes of the last 50 years, especially at the doctor–patient interface, but that is changing with the advent of the Millennial (born 1981–96) and Generation Z (born 1997–2015) groups of clinicians and patients.[1]

Young people born after the advent of the Internet in 1989 are also often referred to as 'digital natives'. This generation was raised in an environment in which living in both real and virtual worlds simultaneously is commonplace and accepted. They want to be able to receive their healthcare in a more accessible and immediate manner, like most other services in their lives. Nakagawa and Yellowlees have documented the differences between the various generations involved in healthcare and the impact that that is having on the use of technology for patient care, across medicine and especially for mental health purposes.[17] They summarised their conclusions as follows:

> Younger physicians will drive technological advancement and integration faster than previous generations, allowing technology to adapt more quickly to serve the needs of clinicians and patients. These changes will improve efficiency, allow more flexible working arrangements, and increase convenience for patients and physicians. The next generation of physicians will use technology to support their work and lifestyle preferences, making them more resilient to burnout than previous generations.

Unfortunately, prior to Covid-19 most technology-related decisions in healthcare were still made by Baby Boomer (born 1946–64) leaders who shepherded the use of faxes, pagers and EHRs and who have had to learn and understand the technologies as they were being developed, rather than being enveloped by them since birth. The experience of Covid-19 has undoubtably accelerated a lot of decision making in the healthcare technology area, and increasingly the younger generations of digital natives are being listened to, and are able to craft policies and champion technologies in healthcare in a very different way from prior generations. This will greatly enhance the use of cyberspace for mental health practice and psychotherapy.[17]

The Global Digital Divide Affects Countries Differently

The 'digital divide' has many components to it, impacting differently in countries around the world, just as Covid-19 has. In Western countries like the United States, Australia and Canada, the main focus of this divide is on internal populations of colour, or racial and ethnic differences, as well as the homeless, poor and aged and those who live in rural or underserved regions, all of whom suffer sometimes massive obstacles as they try to access healthcare either in person or digitally.

Whilst the digital divide has often focused on broadband availability, it can include a wider range of issues from the availability of technology, technology literacy and access to resources such as appropriate insurance coverage to cover digital services, and of course these can all be different across national boundaries and in underdeveloped nations compared with those in the West. It is known that in 'digital deserts', which is how some countries can still be described, patients have decreased healthcare options which can be framed in the larger context of a wide range of social determinants of health. Such digital deserts are characterised by the disproportionate detrimental impact of the divide on the mental health of underserved populations, leading to a vicious cycle of increasing health inequities and disparities within and across countries around the globe. These have greatly accelerated in the last year during the pandemic, adding additional uncertainty about the provision of global mental health services in a number of relatively poorly resourced countries.

The Covid-19 Pandemic and the Global Transformation of Psychiatry

Covid-19 has triggered an unprecedented change in the practice of mental health professionals around the world and has essentially moved the use of health technologies by psychiatrists and other clinical professionals well past the 'tipping point'.[15, 18–20]

The occurrence of the Covid-19 pandemic has dramatically changed the practice of psychiatry in the United States, in particular, but also in many other countries, where regulations have been changed and a rapid series of moves supporting the digital transformation in mental health systems has occurred. These changes are illustrated in the five country 'case studies' presented in this chapter – Australia, Japan, Taiwan, Egypt and Turkey. It is likely that this series of changes will continue, and many will become permanent, as mental health services around the world learn to deal with any 'mental health pandemic' that may follow the Covid-19 pandemic. The use of technology in psychiatric services has become essential to provide care in a time of unpredictable and fluctuating quarantines, and the possibility of long-term societal changes due to required public health measures, including sporadically shutting national borders.

Technology in psychiatry has shifted from a gradual and slowly growing adoption and dissemination to an immediate widespread implementation with dramatic changes in the way that many psychiatrists and other mental health professionals are working around the world. The Covid-19 pandemic will ultimately end and psychiatry will emerge altered by the current dramatic increase in the use of technology and by larger societal trends, especially the move of care direct to the home, and away from clinics and hospitals. Whilst 2021 (the time of writing this chapter) is a time of uncertainty, threat and change, there are massive opportunities to shape and improve global psychiatric systems for the benefit of patients, practitioners and the many diverse populations that psychiatrists serve.[2]

This is best exemplified by the description of the international easing of inhibitory regulations in relation to telepsychiatry post Covid-19 as described by Kinoshita et al.[20] This group of international telepsychiatrists used snowball sampling of 30 collaborators from 17 different countries around the world to report that 13 of the countries had altered telemedicine regulations that had previously restricted the spread of telepsychiatry, at least temporarily initially. The 13 countries that deregulated were Australia, Brazil, Canada, China, Denmark, Germany, India, Italy, Japan, South Africa, South Korea, Taiwan and the United States, whilst the four that did not were Egypt, Spain, Turkey and the UK. Importantly, following these changes in 15 of the regions telepsychiatry consultations were now reimbursed at the same level as in-person consultations, and in all 17 telepsychiatry was now covered by public health insurance, and whilst restrictions on telepsychiatry prescribing were often reduced, they still existed in 11 regions. The authors concluded that these regulation relaxations around the world were likely to lead to a rapid expansion of the use of telepsychiatry and to its extended use.

The following five national 'case studies' have been written by colleagues living in Australia, Japan and Taiwan, where regulation reductions occurred, and in Egypt and Turkey, where they did not.

Australia

In Australia, telepsychiatry has been used in public, private and community settings for consultations, assessments, diagnosis, treatment and even group support or family therapy for more than 30 years. Around one-third of Australians live in rural and remote areas, yet most specialist healthcare services are centralised in large metropolitan regions.

Examples of Australian telepsychiatry services include:

1. *Child and Youth Mental Health Services (CYMHS): eCYMHS is specialist child and youth mental health service established in 2005 and delivered throughout Queensland to support patients living in rural and remote areas.[21]*

2. *eGROW: Grow is a community organisation who, through their eGrow programme, carry out peer support groups via video in order to deliver the well-established Grow programme.[22]*

3. *Call to Mind: This private service is staffed with psychiatrists who can provide consultations by video to anyone in Australia.[23]*

The use of telehealth has been critical during Covid-19. At the start of the pandemic, additional temporary Medicare Benefits Schedule telehealth item numbers were introduced to enable more services to be delivered remotely, therefore reducing the risk of virus transmission amongst patients and staff. At the height of the pandemic in Australia, from April– December 2020, approximately 52% of all mental health-related consultations were provided by telehealth. The challenges of providing telepsychiatry services are the same for most other telehealth services in that a reliable telecommunications infrastructure is required to support remote consultations. In Australia, the National Broadband Network has been a significant investment by the government to deliver high-speed internet services to all Australians and whilst there remain gaps in access to the network due to physical location and/or affordability, further investment is occurring. There is an understanding that telepsychiatry is not solely about technology – it is a new way of doing things. This requires clinicians and patients to learn to adapt whilst ultimately integrating telepsychiatry into routine care.[24]

(Professor A. C. Smith PhD, University of Queensland)

Japan

The first case of Covid-19 was confirmed in Japan in January 2020, and the number of infected people in the country increased since then. As in other countries, the pandemic has had a serious impact on mental health in Japan. As such, telemedicine has become a focus of attention and has been used in part as an infection control measure during the pandemic.

Before the Covid-19 pandemic, telepsychiatry for psychiatric disorders other than dementia and epilepsy was not covered by national health insurance, and the spread of telepsychiatry in Japan had hardly progressed. In 2020, the Ministry of Health, Labor and Welfare deregulated telemedicine on a temporary and exceptional basis,[20] allowing telemedicine to be covered by public insurance in the psychiatric field. However, the prescription of narcotics and psychotropic drugs was not allowed during the first tele-medicine visit, which greatly limited telepsychiatry. The price of telemedicine in Japan has been lower than that of in-person medical services under the national health insurance system for a long time, and although this deregulation has increased the price somewhat, it still remains low. The deregulation has however greatly expanded the use of telemedi-cine in Japan, but despite this many medical institutions are hesitant to introduce it due to the low price. Improvement of the price of national health insurance is an issue for future diffusion in Japan.

(Shotaro Kinoshita and Taishiro Kishimoto, Department of Neuropsychiatry, Keio University School of Medicine, Tokyo, Japan)

Taiwan

Before Covid-19 there was a common national rule for telemedicine, which was regulated by a special law and the guidelines of the Ministry of Health and Welfare, Taiwan. There was a limit to the remote areas in which telemedicine could be provided under the law and the first telemedicine visit was allowed only under three conditions: 1. Specific remote areas; 2. Specific conditions; 3. Life-threatening emergencies. Telemedicine was limited to doctors who were employed by public health centres or specific hospitals where the owners had a contract with the Ministry of Health and Welfare.

After the outbreak of the Covid-19 pandemic, there were step-by-step changes in February, March and April 2020. Firstly, quarantined patients in any areas were allowed to apply for the telemedicine services using a number of commercial apps recommended by Taiwan health bureaus for messaging or videoconferencing. If the Internet was not available, the telephone was allowed for telemedicine consultations, but the voice call had to be recorded. As a provisional measure, telemedicine was allowed even for the first visit, but drug prescription duration was limited to no more than one month.

(Chun-Hung Chang and Kuan-Pin Su, School of Medicine, China Medical University, Taichung, Taiwan)

Egypt

Telepsychiatry started in 2015 through one website,[25] which was designed to provide solutions for psychiatric consultation problems. The online counselling service faced a cultural change problem in a community where a third of the population are illiterate, whilst the rest were not familiar with online counselling, concerned that they will not have the chance to express all their thoughts and feelings to the therapist. Through five years of hard work and overcoming many obstacles, the website became bigger and more popular.

During the Covid-19 pandemic, a dramatic change in knowledge took place within the community regarding online meetings in general and in the medical field in particular. The number of sessions per month taking place on the website doubled, and then tripled in the first two months of the lockdown. This cultural phenomenon enabled other telepsychiatry websites to go live with a range of different user-friendly options. Unfortunately, legislation for e-medicine in services in Egypt is absent. The Ministry of Health in collaboration with the national medical syndicate are trying to write a code of ethics, policies and laws regarding these electronic medical services but writing one year after the start of pandemic, these laws are not yet finalised. (Mohammad ElShami, Co-founder and Medical Advisor, Shezlong telepsychiatry platform)

Turkey

During the pandemic, the Telepsychiatry Section of the Psychiatric Association of Turkey wrote a short guideline about telepsychiatry for psychiatrists and put in on their website. Unfortunately, there were no national changes to regulations designed to ease telepsychiatry during the pandemic; however, citizens were allowed to access all personal health data through a website using the 'e-Nabız' (e-pulse) system established by the Ministry of Health. An online videoconference meeting system, which is called 'Dr. e-Nabız' (Dr. e-Pulse), was also created by the Ministry of Health to provide telehealth services between patients who were Covid-19 positive or who were recently in contact with Covid-19-positive persons, and their physicians.[26]

The use of telepsychiatry during the pandemic has been different across private practices, private hospitals and state hospitals in Turkey. In the private sector use has gone up, but in public hospitals it has been relatively unchanged, except for the enabiz.gov.tr system and for some use with patients who have been diagnosed previously and whose treatment is ongoing. In an unpublished survey of 200 Turkish psychiatrists, 51% of psychiatrists working in private or public hospitals stated that telepsychiatry was used in their institution after the pandemic started (telephone or videoconference) and 33% stated that there had been an increase in the use of telepsychiatry during the pandemic. In addition, 45% stated that they started using telepsychiatry after the pandemic and had not used it previously mainly because of regulatory difficulties.

(Dr Hakan Karaş. Assistant Professor of Psychiatry, İstanbul Gelişim University)

It is in the United States where, arguably, the relaxation of regulations had the greatest numeric impact on numbers of patients seen using telepsychiatry.[18] In March 2020, there were very substantial reductions of inhibitory regulations that had previously adversely impacted reimbursement for video visits and telephony, had constrained consultations via state licensing and geographic restrictions, and had demanded high-level technical security. This deregulation dramatically accelerated telemedicine adoption ensuring that patients and mental health professionals were able to keep physically safe in the new era of social distancing, as described in the 'telepsychiatry toolkit' on the American Psychiatric Association website.[2] At UC Davis Health, where PY works, the psychiatry outpatient service converted from mostly in-person office visits to fully virtual in three days, whilst the rest of the health system converted to a largely virtual operation in one week.[19] A year later in March 2021, with the psychiatry outpatient services still seeing more than 98% of patients virtually, there was no loss of patients, and only half the prior number of 'no-show' appointments, whilst 15–20% of all patients attending medical and surgical outpatient clinics at UC Davis Health continued to be seen on video. Similar stories have been published about other psychiatric services such as Kaiser Permanente, the largest managed care organisation in the United States with 12 million plan members, which moved rapidly to deliver 90% of its psychiatric care virtually.

Suddenly, telepsychiatry became a core healthcare tool for most psychiatrists in the United States.[18] Many clinics rapidly made the move to in-home consultations or virtual house calls. A survey conducted by the American Psychiatric Association during the Covid-19 pandemic found that by June of 2020, 85% of 500 surveyed American psychiatrists were using telepsychiatry, usually video, but with phone as a back-up, with more than 75% of their patients, compared with about 3% prior to Covid-19.2 Yellowlees et al. have detailed the latest available national telehealth statistics derived from 60 US contributing private insurers as at December 2020,[27] which showed an increase of 2,816% in telehealth consultations in all disciplines compared with December 2019, and that these now comprised 6.5% of all consultations nationally, with 47% of the patients being seen for primarily mental health reasons.[28] The National Center for Health Statistics reported a total of 883 million outpatient consultations nationally in the United States in 2018.[29] Projecting from the insurance statistics, Yellowlees and colleagues calculated that about 3% of these in 2020 were telepsychiatry visits (by video or phone), an approximate total of 26 million such visits nationally. An extraordinary increase and whilst it is uncertain as to whether all of these regulatory changes will be permanent, it is likely that many will be, so the conclusion of these authors that there seems no doubt that telepsychiatry has now become a major delivery component of mental health services in the United States is likely correct. Others have noted how apps and other forms of online care rapidly grew more popular in the United States and other countries during the Covid-19 pandemic with Talkspace, an app offering text messages and therapy sessions, reporting a 65% increase in clients since the pandemic started.

In a number of European countries, such as Spain and Italy, technologies like telemedicine were also used to enable altered clinical workflows in response to Covid-19. These included hybrid ward rounds, which became popular with inpatient medical and psychiatric teams divided in space, but connected by video, in order to minimise exposure and use of personal protective equipment. Hybrid rounding has been in practice for quite some time in intensive care units, but Covid-19 expanded this practice across many inpatient services including in psychiatric hospitals, and also enabled services to be conferenced to and from community sites, for example, dialysis or hospice care units, where a number of psychiatrists and other mental health professionals work.

In the United States and elsewhere, Covid-19-related school closures also created an unexpected strain on working parents. The use of telemedicine allowed many clinicians, including some trainee psychiatrists, to work at least part time from home, alleviating some childcare burdens – a move that would have been unimaginable before Covid-19. Such residents were able to continue their training programmes in a hybrid manner, with virtual didactics and mentoring, meetings and social gatherings over video, and regular check-ins and buddy systems via email, phone and text, all rapidly put in place to supplement some core in-person services. These changes driven by Covid-19, literally overnight, promoted teleworking for many clinicians during conventional office hours, and at nights and weekends, a move that was in harmony with generational shifts in needs and attitudes as more millennials became practising clinicians and demanded such choices. At UC Davis prior to the pandemic, all trainee psychiatrists were mandated to see a small proportion of their patients on video, but this all changed when some residents in their outpatient training year literally saw all their patients on video, with psychiatrists providing video supervision, all working from home. Going forward it is planned for trainees to see about half of their outpatients in a hybrid manner, online and in person.

In the United States, many patients have still faced challenges using and accessing video conferencing during Covid-19 due to both comfort and capacity as well as the 'digital divide' as discussed above, but also including healthcare systems' inherent systemic racism.[30] The consequence of this is that Covid-19 has also led to a significant increase in the use of the telephone to manage patients. The literature on psychiatric treatment via telephone prior to the pandemic is limited to structured evidence-based psychotherapies[31] and interactive voice response treatments,[32] and was deficient regarding the ability to complete full psychiatric assessments and conduct treatments via the telephone. A number of studies in the United States are now underway to evaluate the effectiveness of phone consultations, with one large public mental health programme reporting that telephone consultations were highly effective in maintaining a large cohort of inner-city impoverished and racially diverse patients with severe mental illness.[33] In many cases, the clinicians found that telephone visits were more effective than prior in-person visits because there were significantly fewer telephone 'no shows'. Given these results, it would seem that a major silver-lining from Covid-19 might well be the validation of the efficacy of phone consultations by psychiatrists and clinical case managers, especially for groups of patients who are already known to the providers. This has the potential to be another major global change to the practice of psychiatry if other countries follow this US example.

The many novel approaches to hybrid work described above, with more time and geographically flexible working arrangements, will likely lead to long-term workplace solutions that offer psychiatrists increased flexibility and further support the wellbeing of clinicians and their families, allowing them to offer online mental health services literally anytime, anywhere. Suddenly it is no longer unusual for a psychiatrist living and working from home in New York, for example, to be employed part time by a Californian public health system, as well as by one of the now numerous private practice commercial telepsychiatry companies that have commenced practice in the past five years in the United States, seeing patients in other states. No longer are psychiatrists in the United States tied to one place of work, or one set of patients. Instead they are able to take up, if they wish, several different positions, giving them more variety and geographic- and time-related flexibility of professional practice.

International Telepsychiatry Companies

There are hundreds of commercial telepsychiatry companies that offer services within and across national borders around the world. Many of them were originally based in the United States, India, Israel, Australia and Canada as well as the UK, and most of them also offer other medical disciplines, especially primary care, but most estimates in the literature suggest that about half of all telemedicine consultations are for mental health, and this proportion likely increased during the pandemic. It is straightforward to find these companies via Google with simple searches using terms such as 'international telepsychiatry company' and country names. A few of the larger ones are publicly listed and owned, with valuations in billions of dollars, and have been in operation for at least a decade, whilst many more are less than five years old and are not necessarily yet stable. They usually have similar business models consisting of either direct payments for consultations, and/or a 'per member per month' cost, often paid by insurance companies, employee associations or partnering health systems. In recent years, there has been a significant move into this space by major retailers such as Amazon and WalMart,[34] with Google and Microsoft also showing a lot of interest, and it is likely that many of the lessons learned by the retail industry as it has increasingly gone online during the past decade will be applied to healthcare in the next decade. Currently, the single most important barrier for the functioning of these commercial companies is finding enough high-quality clinicians, such as psychiatrists, to work within them, and to provide clinical leadership and quality control, but it is likely that future generations of Millennial and Gen Z psychiatrists will be more prepared to work in such commercial environments than prior generations.

What Have We Learned? Future Directions for Telepsychiatry and the Practice of Psychiatrists

It is clear that there has been a dramatic increase in the amount of telepsychiatry around the world since March 2020. This has led to three major sets of changes to mental health practice that seem likely to be permanent. These are the introduction of hybrid psychiatric care using a range of technologies, the use of virtual home visits, and the move to increase the number and range of asynchronous mental health consultations using a variety of technologies including recorded video.

Innovation 1: Hybrid Psychiatric Care

The use of a 'hybrid' model of care combining in-person consultations and telepsychiatry has been described in detail by Yellowlees and Shore,[1] who defined a hybrid psychiatrist as a clinician who:

> interacts with patients both in-person and online so that their doctor-patient relationship crosses both environments. The addition of interactions via videoconferencing, e-mail, text messaging and telephony leads to improved access and interactions at times and places not possible with care restricted to the in-person venue. This hybrid practice is becoming a preferred model of care for many physicians as secure messaging is incorporated into electronic medical record systems. It is especially relevant to telepsychiatry as a range of video technologies, text-based systems and apps can readily complement in-person care depending on the psychiatrist's and patient's preferences. The incorporation of online models of care into practice can strengthen the doctor-patient relationship by increasing empathy and forming a trusting therapeutic bond. (p. 251)

The American Psychiatric Association has acknowledged how prevalent this style of practice has become amongst American psychiatrists during Covid-19 and published a guidance document as part of their Telepsychiatry Toolkit for members about opening or reopening their practice during Covid-19 (2020) with the following advice:

> the safest way to continue providing treatment is through telehealth when feasible, particularly if this has been a viable option to date. Many patients may want to continue working in a hybrid way, with a mix of in-person and telehealth visits.[2]

It is likely that in the post-Covid-19 world, many, if not most, mental health professionals will continue to practise in this hybrid manner, seeing patients both online and in person, depending on mutual convenience and preference. This may well lead to the development of several novel future psychotherapies and mental health treatments that will take the best aspects of both in-person and online models of care and therapy and combine them. In some places this is already happening, with Fortney et al. describing the use of online video sessions with veterans who have PTSD as an engagement strategy to eventually lead to them attending in-person group sessions.[35] Box 7.1 is an example of the current practice of hybrid psychiatry.

Box 7.1 Case study: the hybrid psychiatrist

PY has taken advantage of the dramatic improvements in mobile devices and no longer owns a desktop computer, nor does he have a fixed telephone line to his home. During Covid-19, he has seen all his patients at home. He uses three wireless mobile devices for all his professional and personal activities – a laptop, iPad and iPhone – with a large computer screen that any of these devices can be plugged into if preferred. Figure 7.1 is a photograph of his home desk where all patient activities occur. PY uses three types of videoconferencing with patients (Extended Care via Epic, Zoom and Webex) and has three differing versions of the Epic electronic medical record (Epic, Haiku and Canto), available on his three mobile devices all connected via apps or a virtual private network to UC Davis Health servers. He has access to secure direct messaging with patients via the Electronic Medical Record (EMR), as well as secure email and messaging to colleagues and patients as required. He is able to use telepsychiatry to see patients and supervise residents, often situated in three different home environments at once, whilst using apps for education, therapy and remote monitoring. He sees patients on real-time (synchronous) video in Indian Health primary care clinics around California, in their homes via the UC Davis outpatient department and in nursing homes. He sees other patients using asynchronous methods – either asynchronous telepsychiatry with pre-recorded video consultations, or e-consults performed in the electronic medical record giving opinions on treatment options for requesting primary care physicians. He also performs occasional pro-bono asynchronous messaged provider-to-provider e-consults for a charity to primary care clinics around the world in places like Bangladesh, Nigeria, India and Nepal. Prior to Covid-19, all his outpatients were managed in a hybrid manner, being seen in-person or online depending on his, and their, choice and convenience, and it is likely that post-Covid-19 he will return to this practice, although he expects to do proportionately many fewer in-person consultations over time.

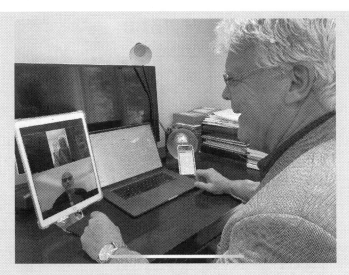

Figure 7.1 The hybrid psychiatrist at work

Innovation 2: The Return of the Virtual Home Visit

The introduction of smartphones and mobile devices as described previously has suddenly made it possible to easily connect with patients direct in their homes, their workplaces, social environments and their vehicles, rather than having to see them in primary care clinics as has been the case with traditional telepsychiatry. This has revolutionised the practice of telemental health, especially following the adaptation of American Telemedicine Association guidelines for delivering video mental healthcare at home or in community settings.[5] These guidelines importantly included standard operating procedures to ensure patient safety in community settings and have been widely adopted by telepsychiatry practitioners around the world.

At the time of writing this chapter, one year into the Covid-19 pandemic, most US-based telepsychiatrists now deliver care direct to patients in non-clinical community settings routinely. The home offers many more opportunities to get to know patients and to further deepen understanding and the level of the doctor–patient relationship. Yellowlees and Shore have described the process of the virtual home visit as follows:[15]

> It is possible to take a tour of the home and garden, and thereby discover a patient's interests in art, from pictures on the walls, or sports, from memorabilia on counters. Equally it is possible to see how a patient lives more easily than if only meeting them in a clinic. Is their home neat and tidy, or chaotic? Do they have personal space? Do they have pets, and how do they look after them? What about others in the family? Can you speak to parents, partners, children, and perhaps get a better idea of the patient's relationships, and the views of people important in their lives about how the patient is coping. Does the patient have food in the house? Are there a surprising number of bottles of alcohol in evidence? Is

there a suggestion of disorganization, with unwashed plates in the kitchen, and dirty clothes on the floor? Does the patient have a sense of pride and commitment to their home, and are they interested in gardening, and prepared to show you around not just the house, but the garden and immediate locality to give you more of an idea of how and where they live? (p. 103)

There are several specific advantages of seeing patients on video in their homes or community settings. These include:

- The doctor–patient relationship is likely more egalitarian, and the environment is less intimidating for patients.
- The interview can be more intimate, especially when trauma is involved, as the slightly increased virtual distance frequently makes it easier for patients to confide in their physician.
- The consultation is more convenient and safer for both parties, who both save both time and cost – physicians can type notes at the same time as maintaining eye contact with their patient and also save time by not having to physically move patients in and out of their room.
- There is less stigma and fear and no need for a patient to be physically seen in a psychiatry clinic.
- Fewer 'no shows' and can talk the patient through technology issues via the phone.
- Teamwork is easier, with the ability to bring in other relatives, providers or colleagues.
- More information can be found in the home setting which is really an extension of the mental state exam – homes are a reflection of who we are.
- More people such as family, carers and supporters can be involved, as long as there is privacy awareness.
- More insight can be developed about a patient's interests and passions, from grandchildren to pets, hobbies and gardens.
- Specific findings are possible by looking for the presence of alcohol, the contents of refrigerators and general cleanliness.
- All of these positives lead to improved provider wellbeing and patient satisfaction.

The potential disadvantages compared to in-person consultations are the same as for most telepsychiatry consultations, namely:

- Some patients and physicians have anxiety and phobias, or ignorance, about technology, or cannot afford it, and patients who are homeless or seriously mentally ill may not have access.
- Some physicians complain of 'Zoom fatigue' if doing too many video sessions, but this can be resolved by taking breaks and not booking sessions completely back to back.
- Some physicians complain of a loss of 'in-person feel' and capacity to understand the patient so well, but this usually resolves over time.
- Aspects of the psychiatrically relevant physical exams can be difficult, but patients can buy most equipment needed for vital sign measurement, and tests such as the Abnormal Involuntary Movements Scale can be assessed online.
- Privacy is always a concern, and it is important to confirm who is in the home and that doors are shut, or that the patient is comfortable with the privacy level. In cars, patients need to be aware that they can often be heard through closed windows in parking garages if they speak loudly.

Innovation 3: Asynchronous Telepsychiatry

Yellowlees et al. have recently reported on a two-year randomised clinical trial of synchronous telepsychiatry compared with asynchronous telepsychiatry in primary care patients and have found that both modalities led to similarly improved clinical outcomes.[27] The authors noted that asynchronous telepsychiatry can be a more data-rich form of the traditional medical or psychiatric consultation and described the process whereby a trained interviewer conducts and records a semi-structured interview with the patient, which is combined with other available clinical data such as from electronic medical records. This recorded video consult and information from the EMR is made accessible to a telepsychiatrist who reviews it before providing an opinion on the patient's diagnosis and treatment options. Early pilot studies in the United States, Canada and India provide evidence that asynchronous video consultations have similar diagnostic accuracy to synchronous telepsychiatry in English and across languages (where interpreted subheadings are added to the video), that it is a feasible consultation modality in primary care patients and with patients cared for in skilled nursing facilities, and that it may also be less costly to implement.

The interest in asynchronous telepsychiatry is primarily because, despite the success of real-time video visits, or synchronous telepsychiatry, which is now the current standard international telepsychiatry practice as described above, administrative and technical challenges with it exist, especially around scheduling of telepsychiatrists and patients.[1,36–38] Importantly from an international perspective, synchronous telepsychiatry itself is simply a virtual extension of in-person care which cannot be scaled to enable one physician to see more patients. Asynchronous care makes use of a completely virtual care model with the potential to scale, with psychiatrists consulting on more patients per hour than if they were seeing them all personally. This enables psychiatrists to be more efficiently involved in the treatment of more patients over a given time period, just as occurs with the charity work described above where, instead of the data reviewed being video clips, it is usually photographs of case notes. As such it is of great potential interest in countries around the world where psychiatrists are in short supply. In recent years, asynchronous technologies have become more widespread in many healthcare settings, and especially in radiology, dermatology, ophthalmology, cardiology and pathology, and such asynchronous tools have been expanding into mental healthcare where they may be at least a partial solution to address the psychiatrist workforce shortage and reduce access barriers for patients.[1] Other positive patient outcomes have been demonstrated with e-coaching for depression,[39] mobile based asynchronous text-messaging therapy with a licensed therapist[40] and with an integrated asynchronous virtual care platform.[41]

Conclusions

It is evident that the practice of telepsychiatry, using not just real-time videoconferencing, but a wide range of technologies and synchronous and asynchronous approaches to mental healthcare, is expanding rapidly around the world. There is no doubt that the Covid-19 pandemic has had an enormous impact and has pushed the implementation of such online mental health systems in many countries well past the 'tipping point' so that it is likely that in the post-pandemic world they will be increasingly integrated into all forms of mental healthcare delivery.

Most telepsychiatry is still delivered within national boundaries, with often very different approaches to regulation, but a number of cross-national companies and charities are emerging that will further shrink the practice of psychiatry around the world, making psychiatrists more accessible to patients and hopefully providing more effective models of hybrid mental healthcare direct to patients' homes and communities, anytime, anywhere. It is likely that asynchronous models of care will significantly expand, driven by younger generations of both physicians and patients, as well as by psychiatrist shortages and the improvements in devices and technological solutions. It is evident that the biggest international barrier to telepsychiatry that still remains in many countries is excessive inhibitory regulations, and these need to be reduced if the hybrid mental health services and approaches to care described here are to be effectively implemented in the future.

References

1. Yellowlees, P., Shore, J. *Telepsychiatry and Health Technologies: A Guide for Mental Health Professionals*. Washington DC: APPI Press. 2018.

2. American Psychiatric Association. n.d. APA Telepsychiatry Toolkit. Available at: www.psychiatry.org/psychiatrists/practice/telepsychiatry (accessed 3 April 2021).

3. Yellowlees, P., Chan, S. R., Parish, M. The hybrid doctor–patient relationship in the age of technology: telepsychiatry consultations and the use of virtual space. *Int. Rev. Psychiatry*. 2015;27(6): 476–89.

4. Chan, S., Li, L., Torous, J., Gratzer, D., Yellowlees, P. M. Review of use of asynchronous technologies incorporated in mental health care. *Curr. Psychiatry Rep*. 2018;20(10): 85. https://doi.org/10.1007/s1 1920-018-0954-3.

5. Shore, J. H., Yellowlees, P., Caudill, R. et al. Best practices in videoconferencing-based telemental health April 2018. *Telemed. J. E. Health*. 2018;24(11): 827–32.

6. Bashshur, R., Shannon, G., Bashshur, N., Yellowlees, P. The empirical evidence for telemedicine interventions in mental disorders. *Telemed. J. E. Health*. 2016;22(2): 87–113.

7. Hilty, D., Ferrer, D., Parish, M. B., Johnston, B., Callahan, E., Yellowlees, P. The effectiveness of telemental health: a 2013 review. *Telemed. J. E. Health*. 2013;19(6): 444–54.

8. American Telemedicine Association. n.d. Available at: www.americantelemed.org (accessed 3 April).

9. International Society for Telemedicine and eHealth. n.d. Available at: www.isfteh.org (accessed 3 April 2021).

10. Shore, J. H. Managing virtual hybrid psychiatrist–patient relationships in a digital world. *JAMA Psychiatry*. 2020;77 (5): 541–2.

11. Chan, S., Torous, J., Hinton, L., Yellowlees, P. Towards a framework for evaluating mobile mental health apps. *Telemed. J. E. Health*. 2015;21(12): 1038–41.

12. Chan, S., Parish, M., Yellowlees, P. Telepsychiatry today. *Curr. Psychiatry Rep*. 2015;17(11): 89.

13. Deyan. G. 67+ revealing smartphone statistics for 2020. *Techjury*. 31 July 2020. Available at: https://techjury.net/blog/smartphone-usage-statistics/%23gref. (accessed 3 April 2021).

14. Yellowlees, P., Chan, S. R. Mobile mental health care: an opportunity for India. *Indian J. Med. Res*. 2015;142(4): 359–61.

15. Yellowlees, P., Shore J. *Psychotherapy in Cyberspace*. In Crisp, H., Gabbard, G. O., eds., *Gabbard's Textbook of Psychotherapeutic Treatments*. Washington, DC: American Psychiatric Publishing. 2023. pp. 719–41.

16. Yellowlees, P. M., Holloway, K. M., Parish, M. B. Therapy in virtual environments–clinical and ethical issues. *Telemed. J. E. Health*. 2012;18(7): 558–64.

17. Nakagawa, K., Yellowlees, P. Inter-generational effects of technology: why millennial physicians may be less at risk for

burnout than baby boomers.*Curr. Psychiatry Rep.* 2020;22(9): 45.

18. Shore, J. H., Schneck, C. D., Mishkind, M. C. Telepsychiatry and the coronavirus disease 2019 pandemic: current and future outcomes of the rapid virtualization of psychiatric care. *JAMA Psychiatry.* 2020;77(12):1211–2. https://doi .org/10.1001/jamapsychiatry.2020.1643.

19. Yellowlees, P., Nakagawa, K., Pakyurek, M., Hanson, A., Elder, J., Kales, H. Rapid conversion of an outpatient psychiatric clinic to a 100% virtual telepsychiatry clinic in response to COVID-19. *Psychiatr. Serv.* 2020;71(7): 749–52.

20. Kinoshita, S., Cortright, K., Crawford, A., Mizuno, Y. et al. Changes in telepsychiatry regulations during the COVID-19 pandemic: 17 countries and regions' approaches to an evolving healthcare landscape. *Psychol. Med.* 2020;52(13): 1–8. https://doi.org/10.1017/ S0033291720004584.

21 Queensland Government. Child and Youth Mental Health Service community clinics. n.d. Available at: www.childrens.health.qld .govau/service-mental-health-community- clinics/ (accessed 3 April 2021).

22. GROW. eGrow Group. 2020. Available at: https://grow.org.au/egrow/ (accessed 29 March 2021).

23. Call to Mind. 2021. Available at: https:// calltomind.com.au/ (accessed 29 March 2021).

24. Thomas, E. E., Haydon, H. M., Mehrotra, A. et al. Building on the momentum: sustaining telehealth beyond COVID-19. *J. Telemed. Telecare.* 2020; Sep 26: 1357633X20960638. https://doi .org/10.1177/1357633X20960638. Epub ahead of print.

25. Shezlong Counseling website. n.d. Available at: www.shezlong.com (accessed 5 April 2021).

26. Dr e-Pulse website. n.d. Available at: https://dr.enabiz.gov.tr (accessed 5 April 2021).

27. Yellowlees, P., Parish, M., Gonzalez, A. et al. Clinical outcomes of asynchronous

v synchronous telepsychiatry in primary care: a randomized controlled trial. *JMIR.* July 2021;23(7). www.jmir.org/2021/7/e24 047/.

28. Fair Health. Monthly Telehealth Regional Tracker, Dec. 2020. 2020. Available at: htt ps://s3.amazonaws.com/media2 .fairhealth.org/infographic/telehealth/dec- 2020-national-telehealth.pdf (accessed 4 March 2021).

29. National Center for Health Statistics. Ambulatory care use and physician office visits. 2020. Available at: www.cdc.gov/ nchs/fastats/physician-visits.htm. (accessed 4 March 2021).

30. Ramsetty, A., Adams, C. Impact of the digital divide in the age of Covid-19. *JAMIA.* 2020;27(7): 1147–8.

31. Everitt, H. A., Landau, S., O'Reilly, G. et al. . Assessing telephone-delivered CBT and web-delivered CBT versus treatment as usual in irritable bowel syndrome: a multicenter randomized trial. *Gut.* 2019;68(9): 1613–23.

32. Rose, G. L., Badger, G. J., Skelly, J. M. et al. A randomized controlled trial of brief intervention by interactive voice response. *Alcohol Alcohol.,*2017;52(3): 335–43.

33. Avalone, L., Barron, C., King, C. et al. Rapid telepsychiatry implementation during COVID-19: increased attendance at the largest health system in the United States. *Psychiatr. Serv.* 2021;72 (6): 708–11.

34. Nakagawa, K., Yellowlees, P. Retail outlets using telehealth pose significant policy questions for health care. *Health Aff.* 2018;37(12): 2069–75.

35. Fortney, J. C., Pyne, J. M., Turner, E. E. et al. Telepsychiatry integration of mental health services into rural primary care settings. *Int. Rev. Psychiatry.* 2015;27(6): 525–39.

36. Yellowlees, P., Odor, A., Parish, M. et al. Asynchronous telepsychiatry for psychiatric consultations. *Psychiatr. Serv.* 2010;61(8): 375–8.

37. Yellowlees, P. Odor, A, Parish, M. B. Cross-lingual asynchronous

telepsychiatry: disruptive innovation? *Psychiatr. Serv.* 2012;63(9): 945–6.

38. Yellowlees, P., Burke Parish, M., González, A. et al. Asynchronous telepsychiatry: a component of stepped integrated care. *Telemed. J. E. Health.* 2018; 24(5): 375–8.

39. Baumeister, H., Reichler, L., Munzinger, M., Lin, J. The impact of guidance on Internet-based mental health interventions: a systematic review. *Internet Interv.* 2014;1(4): 205–15.

40. Hull, T. D., Mahan, K. A study of asynchronous mobile-enabled SMS text psychotherapy. *Telemed. eHealth.* 2017;23 (3): 240–7.

41. Melmed, A. Chat with a doctor: using asynchronous virtual care access for on-demand physician advice. *iProc.* 2017;3 (1): e18.

Chapter

8

The Integration Agenda
Getting Everything Joined Up

Rob Waller and James Reed

No man is an island entire of itself;
  every man is a piece of the continent, a piece of the main.
John Donne, 1624[1]

The quote above is almost too well known but applies as well to this topic as to anything else. Your new shiny Electronic Health Record (EHR) does not exist in isolation. Those who use our service exist outside of it and have data trails there too – many of which are mental health related.

A key driver for integration is because sharing information [securely] improves the care we deliver and patient safety. Dame Fiona Caldicott, a leader in the field of patient confidentiality, introduced the seventh Caldicott Principle in 2013: 'The duty to share information can be as important as the duty to protect patient confidentiality.'[2] Sharing should also occur because service users usually expect us to have shared it already and are annoyed when we don't and they have to repeat themselves, especially if the topic is traumatic for them.[*] We also want to share because we can, but technology itself is not (some would say *should* not be) the prime mover here.

Box 8.1 shows something of what interoperability can do. Much of this has been brought online as the result of rapid digitisation during 2020 as a result of the Covid-19 pandemic, but some rough corners still need smoothing off and it needs extending out to partner organisations and mental health services

We will cover why systems don't seem to talk well to each other, how they can do so securely and ethically and how progress is being made. We are a long way from being able to call up everything about a person with a few clicks of the mouse, and this is probably a good thing, but we do want to be able to access the right information at the right time – to deliver better care.

---

[*] Whilst there is no formal research on this and it is not one of the six key principles of trauma-informed care, the authors have heard multiple accounts of service users who have been needlessly distressed when asked for details of their past traumas when (a) they have already told someone else in the organisation this and (b) it is not necessary for the decision at hand. Better electronic records that can securely record and appropriately make summaries available should reduce this, meaning information only needs to be briefly reviewed and does not have to be disclosed as if for the first time and so retraumatise the service user.

> **Box 8.1** What 'good' looks like
>
> Imagine that your 80-year-old aunt has fallen at home and that we have good systems of interoperability. The call-button round her neck that she presses is able to call for an ambulance, but also alert her social worker that her regular care package will need to be put on hold. The ambulance staff who attend can see that she is a Type 2 diabetic, has a dementia diagnosis and that a power of attorney lies with her daughter, for whom a phone number is given. On admission, her current list of medicines from her GP can be accessed, along with an alert about allergic reactions to some anaesthetics.
>
> On discharge, the named social worker is automatically contacted by the ward team to restart her care package and the social worker can see relevant medical information to commission short-term additional care. Her GP is informed of changes to medications automatically, with extra checks for them and the discharging doctor against the admission medications. The GP and daughter can join a video review with the practice nurse at the patient's house a week later. The local dementia third-sector organisation is informed of the admission and arrange to visit her.

Disintegrated by Design

This fragmentation has arisen for several reasons. Many current systems grew out of 'PAS' systems (Patient Administration Systems) whose primary focus was tracking activity, bed occupancy and referrals. It was hard enough for different parts of the organisation to communicate, let alone think about joining up the dots with those outside!

It was only later that clinical information began to get added. Sometimes, this was to augment the PAS platform. Other attempts started in 'easy win' areas like digitising prescription charts which, to be fair, did often have systems for sending a discharge letter to a GP digitally, but not much more. Piecemeal politically driven funding for specific projects (like a patient-held record) would see only certain types of connectivity focused on.

One analogy is to think of a modern newly built hospital. Everything seems to be arranged logically until someone realises an MRI scanner is needed, so this is bolted on the side. Then a discharge lounge; next a regional unit is located there. Eventually, the whole site is a maze with apocryphal stories of medical students disappearing for days at a time. The question is whether to tear the whole lot down and build again, or to keep on trying to add on as logically as possible.

The current 'smorgasbord' of IT systems in healthcare is like this ageing hospital. Whilst it would be nice to tear it all down and build from scratch, this is not going to happen. The recent direction of travel has been to try and add things on sensibly but increasingly there is a drive to think outside the box. Data can be separated from software, code to safety share information can be written and the patient can be put back at the centre. It's their data after all . . .

The Wachter Report recommended to 'build in interoperability from the start'.[3] This may not be there at the moment, but those who commission healthcare can mandate the ability to share and how it should be done.

Who Needs to Know?

When we speak to our colleagues in the IT department to ask if such and such can be done, the usual reply is that anything is possible if you have enough in your budget. This is not 100% true, but it is accurate that the technical ability to share is rarely the limiting factor.

What's much harder is deciding *what* to share and with *whom* – discussions that start with an understanding of *why* we need to share. Various stakeholders have legitimate places at the table. These people all want data for some legitimate and often legal reasons.

- Secondary care hospitals and clinics – the data they share is largely for internal use but some does need to be shared
- GPs and primary care – drawing together information from different secondary care providers and also delivering lots of care locally
- Social care and other statutory bodies – who legitimately need some information
- Third-sector partners – who need information to deliver services
- Unscheduled care – ambulance, police, especially out of hours or out of area
- The service user – it's their data according to many data rules
- 'Managers' – a catch-all term for those who strategically count, plan and pay
- Researchers – who want to study patterns and trends

Increasingly we are discovering that appropriate sharing of data saves lives, improves staff and service user experience and make services more efficient. Some examples are:

- A service user attends in an emergency out of hours to find that what is already known about them is easily available to the assessing clinician, meaning they don't need as long an assessment, don't have to disclose (again!) their traumatic past and don't have to remember exactly what medication they are on. Instead, they can focus on why they need help now and coming up with a suitable plan.
- A clinician in the above scenario can see (via a short summary) what has gone on in recent therapy sessions that might have been difficult, that there is an appointment in two days that the service user had forgotten about and that the social worker has recently approved additional community support. Admission, including use of the Mental Health Act, is avoided.
- A service user feels more involved in their recovery by receiving letters automatically, ordering repeat medication digitally and being able to submit patient-reported outcomes so they only need clinician input if things are deteriorating.
- A national strategy to manage how lockdown measures are released in the Covid-19 pandemic is informed by near-live data from multiple sources including hospitals, GPs, labs (some private)] and mobile-phone apps.

This is not without its challenges, however. A common thorny issue is the consent model used. Is consent assumed and implied (which many service users assume is the case), trusting that what is shared is only what needs to be shared? Or is it explicit, with nothing shared unless a box has been actively ticked (which is what some service users and some human rights groups want)? A survey of NHS mental health service users found that almost 90% were willing to share both mental health and physical health data[4] – however, how does a system manage those who want to opt out? Similarly, information governance legislation in the UK allows for quite extensive sharing of information for essential healthcare purposes – but this is a broad term that does not always align with what people think is being

> **Box 8.2** The Great North Care Record and consent
>
> This is a read-only shared record across much of north-east England and has a well-thought-through consent policy. They have this built into their data model and it controls who has access to various types of data. They have moved away from a 'permission to view model' (where they have to ask each time) to a presumed-consent model.[5] This is because, with wider sharing, the patient is not always sat in front of you. Legally, this is an acceptable way to use the information, as people can opt out and request the information held. Data is stored centrally on an Information Sharing Gateway.[†] However, they also take the view 'that it's nice manners to ask' and they now routinely ask people to opt in to sending more of their record to university research partners.

shared. The Great North Care Record is a good example of a consent model – as explained in Box 8.2.

Another issue is data overload. We have gone from being data poor to data rich and swapped one set of problems for another. There is so much information in hospital systems now that it can be hard to know when you have had 'a good enough look'; then consider adding in feeds from outside . . . Chapter 5 in this book on artificial intelligence provides one answer, but we are not there yet.

Related to this is the question of where the 'master' record lives – if someone has two addresses, do you believe the one in the GP record or the hospital record? One trite reply is to let the patient edit the record – though organisations have understandable nerves about this.

Standard Setting

Computers, just like humans, need to share a language to communicate effectively. Many readers will be familiar with HTTP and HTTPS (hypertext transfer protocol – secure) that describe much of how internet pages work. More recent developments allow healthcare information to be coded and stored; however, it's not always straightforward.

Dr Bob Wachter, whose report we quoted above, uses the analogy of taking money out of an ATM or bank machine.[6] If you want £100 cash, you can get it out of a machine at your own bank, but also out of many other machines. This is because £100 is a clearly understood unit – one bank just tells the other that the withdrawal has been made. However, sharing medical information is more complex. A simple-sounding concept like 'Depression' needs refining to something like a severe ongoing depression, which could then be coded as '6A71 Recurrent depressive disorder' in ICD-11 but '296.33 Major Depressive Disorder' in DSM-V. Beyond diagnosis, concepts like 'distress' or 'trauma' or 'homeless' are even harder to pin down.

Before considering some recent and current developments later in the chapter, it is helpful to outline some principles. The Healthcare Information and Management Systems Society, Inc. (HIMSS) suggest four levels of planning before this sort of communication can take place.[7]

[†] www.informationsharinggateway.org.uk/

1. **Foundation**: That the systems can 'see' each other in the digital landscape. This requires organisations to have at least some external visibility of their databases from outside their firewall.
2. **Structure**: How the data flows and where does it live on the way. New computer languages can perform a 'digital handshake' to make sure the right systems are connected, but legislation requires careful consideration of any pooling of data on the way. For example: an overseas server is often seen as unacceptable due to different data laws in that country.
3. **Semantic**: There are language standards – the £100 analogy about making sure the systems understand each other and put things in similar places. (SNOMED-CT is a more well-known example.) There are also interface standards (called APIs – application programming interfaces) that describe how groups of similar data types should look.
4. **Organisational**: This is about the highest and often most hard-to-sort level. Even if there are more technical solutions to levels 1–3, there need to be policies and consent models, build up in an atmosphere of trust and subject to regular review.

A delicate balance is needed when attempting to legislate or control this area. It is tempting to take a top-down approach and mandate what should be shared, but there are lessons to be learned from the United States 'Meaningful Use' programme.[‡] What started as a desire to share became a requirement to share in order to tick a box to receive Medicare funding or claim for insurance and now sees millions of pieces of data shared everyday into the ether with little prospect of them ever being used. Closer to home in the UK, central planners have always wanted reports and data. However, the list of things that now must be reported on is very long,[§] with things added all the time – and little taken off the list.[**]

Making Connections

The story of healthcare systems' communication with each other starts with some notable failures. Driven by powerful arguments such as medical errors being the third leading cause of *preventable* death worldwide,[8] it was decided that making clinical information available to clinicians was the way to change this. Whilst some small local systems did this well, an early attempt to do so on a larger scale was the Department of Health's National Program for IT (NPfIT) described in detail in Chapter 1. It was too centralised to work.

This is a tricky area to work in. Challenges include:

- Health and social care is big, decentralised and risk-averse.
- Digital underinvestment with many legacy (old, unsupported) systems.
- Standards that were adopted were poorly developed, not robustly implemented or not well tracked.

[‡] The 'Meaningful Use' programme is now called the 'Medicare Promoting Interoperability Program' and encourages healthcare providers in the United States to adopt, implement, upgrade and meaningfully use electronic health records. More information is available at www.cms.gov/regula tions-and-guidance/legislation/ehrincentiveprograms?redirect=/ehrincentiveprograms/30_mean ingful_use.asp (accessed 20 June 2023).
[§] This is the current list of what the Department of Health in England wants to collect: https://digital .nhs.uk/data-and-information/data-collections-and-data-sets/data-collections
[**] This is contentious and not easy to find a published reference for. We would recommend readers ask their local data office whether the list of requirements is getting shorter or longer.

Clinically led standards around communication have been developed in the UK by the Professional Records Standards Body.[††] These are clear and ethical standards based on the principles of good communication and contain valuable headings for information such as in their Mental Health Inpatient Discharge Summary Standards.[‡‡] However, until very recently, they had not been written in a way that computers can understand and so have not been adopted by any of the major EHR vendors.

Keeping It Simple

Better attempts to join things up on a large scale have been to keep it simple. In the UK, the concept of the 'NHS number' has existed for many decades, but was not embedded into IT systems. Many local hospitals had their own number, often taken from paper casenotes which were generated on an 'as needed' basis. The Scottish version, the 'CHI number' (Community Health Index) was the first to be routinely used for digital health communications and is being developed as a unique number across social care as well.[§§] South of the border, the NHS number now sits firmly at the centre of digital healthcare and has enabled many of the initiatives described in the following sections. Some countries have resisted a national number, often for reasons of civil liberties, but are now increasingly envious of the UK.

Picking the Low-Hanging Fruit

One area of healthcare that lends itself to digitisation is medicines management – often through an ePMA (electronic prescribing and medicines administration) system. Medication doses and names are relatively stable. ePMAs were often the vanguard through which hospitals started using an EHR, with the ePMA generating the discharge letter. However, even with something as granular as medication, there are still different naming conventions used, which is a major reason why the big benefits of medicines reconciliation are yet to be fully realised.

Integration by Design

One approach is to go back to the drawing board and get the data architecture right before you build any clinical systems. This 'integration by design' means being clear about where your data lives and how it flows and communicates, and then expecting various digital solutions to base themselves on this.

This is something of a purists' approach, which can seem to ignore the current state of play and the vast amounts of healthcare data already in play. However, a simple understanding of data architecture will help us design good and interoperable systems.

Figure 8.1 shows the two main ways data can be stored. In the first example, most data is held within large software programs based in GP surgeries or hospitals. They do share data, but only for specific things. A good recent example is lots of healthcare organisations sharing their data on Covid-19-positive patients to a central database. In the second example, the data is stored at a central level and suitably tagged so the 'top level' (the software clinicians actually work with) draws on it.

[††] https://theprsb.org/   [‡‡] https://theprsb.org/standards/mentalhealth/
[§§] Extract from the Public Health Scotland data dictionary: www.ndc.scot.nhs.uk/Dictionary-A-Z/ Definitions/index.asp?ID=128 (accessed 21 March 2022).

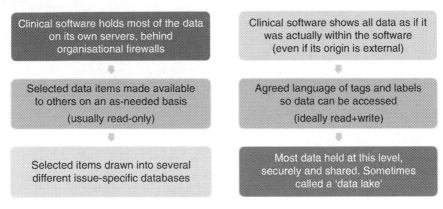

Figure 8.1 Two types of data architecture

The key thing is the middle level – the language used to share. However, the second arrangement requires widespread development. It's like writing a dictionary for all of health and social care and then all agreeing what the definitions are. This might sound tricky, but a similar situation exists with the internet encyclopedia called Wikipedia. Here, someone starts an entry, but others can come in and clarify it, subdivide it and add to it.*** The same type of 'open source' development is described in Box 8.3.

Box 8.3 OpenEHR

This is an organic system for describing data in health and social care that anyone can access and contribute to. For example, within a dataset for mental health, a 'community team' dataset could be created. New roles could be added, and new status (keyworker, assistant, etc.). Each item has an associated FHIR (Fast Healthcare Interoperability Resources) code. (The next section explains more about FHIR.)

Once created, this 'community mental health team' dataset is available for anyone to use. As a result, apps like the Chart-My-Health app can be designed to receive both inputs from service users but also link into the hospitals records in a meaningful way.††† Service users can choose their keyworker from a live list and share their data with them. This promotes service-user engagement, ownership of recovery and joint working. The main thing is that in a sense OpenEHR is not about interoperability at all but about building systems that do not need interoperability since the apps are built to work against a common data platform and common data definitions.

The key message here is that data architecture systems like OpenEHR are not about interoperability at all but about building systems that do not need interoperability since the apps are built to work against a common data platform and common data definitions. Everyone gets to play.

*** https://en.wikipedia.org/wiki/Wikipedia:About ††† https://chartmyhealth.apperta.org

The Wachter Report (Recommendation 9) recommended building in interoperability from the start, but they were not recommending actually starting from scratch – instead, it was more about having some core standards and enforcing them, and allowing a mixed ecosystem so that no one vendor (EHR provider) dominates. In the same way that the 'Big Five' (Amazon, Microsoft, Google, Apple and Facebook) dominate much of everyday technology, healthcare can be dominated by some big names who can be data greedy, wanting to keep all the data on their systems and not share.

There is also something of a 'chicken and egg' scenario here. If the big vendors don't share their data, then there will be no 'little guys' coming in to be creative and drive competition; however, without these smaller companies, no one wants or needs the architecture. However, other healthcare systems internationally (mainly the United States, see Chapter 7) have seen multiple small companies creating good products that clinicians and others now want to integrate. A key enabler has been the willingness of governments to fund national (or regional) data platforms where the 'data lake' can be stored securely but with public ownership too.

A Diverse Ecosystem

The realists' approach is to see that whilst much data is currently tied up in large-scale EHRs (sometimes called 'enterprise systems'), there is also a growing need to share. Because much of the data in enterprise systems is very organisation specific (e.g. what ward someone is on and which bed on that ward and why the bed next to them is closed), it doesn't need to be shared and is often badly coded anyway.

This means that the focus is on coding what needs to be shared with other systems. Previously in this chapter, we used the analogy of £100 being shared between banks as simple, but sharing more nuanced terms as more tricky. The mechanisms for getting data from one place to another and structuring the request are now starting to be described using languages like HL7 and FHIR. Clinicians don't need to know the language, but it can be helpful to know that a request of 'Tell me the current diagnosis' will have a different FHIR code from 'Tell me the current medications' or 'Tell me the last appointment date in surgery'.

As you can imagine, the lists of these codes quickly get very big, but because they are publicly held on accessible platforms, they can be seen by all software developers and allow information to be shared in a secure way. Increasingly, the large enterprise systems are building FHIR into their software so they can (in theory) share information. The Great North Care Record mentioned earlier in this chapter is one example of where this has happened to some degree, but there are many (including service users) who want more to be shared, but are struggling to get progress.

Compounding this is that the companies who make some of the large enterprise systems have also developed data lakes – data repositories that they control. They can do amazing things with their data in these interfaces, but it can be hard for other developers to get in on the act and of course competition is not something they want to directly encourage!

CareConnect APIs

This technical term actually describes something that might be a halfway house to solve this problem. The NHS in England have developed a fairly detailed set of FHIR-coded terms that have been developed with extensive patient and clinician testing that are now required interfaces for all software that NHS England runs. These 'APIs' must also be turned 'on' and not hidden away until the right financial lever appears.

What this will mean over time is that information is more freely available to all developers who can work with FHIR, which is a secure language suitable for healthcare. You will no longer need one system for the whole hospital or organisation – separate systems should be able to easily pass information. For example, the digital prescribing system will pass information into the mental health system, which in turn can pass it to a GP system. You could also have one system with an intuitive interface sitting over several systems that do the heavy lifting – one example is Miya Precision.‡‡‡ This also encourages innovation and competition by definition – sometimes another enterprise system and sometimes a small start-up or even a patient-held app. This is being coordinated by an 'Open API Policy'.[9]

To kick-start the implementation of this, some parts of England were given additional funding as LHCREs (Local Health and Care Record Exemplar) and more recently as 'Shared Care Records'. There have been some regional records developed and they have been shown to be a good idea to both service users and politicians, but things are still a long way from the kinds of thing that interoperability could deliver. New initiatives such as Integrated Care Systems may be able to take this further, bringing a requirement to work together and the statutory changes needed to get round complicated data ownership.[10]

Patient Portals

If you can send data to a GP or social worker, you can also send it to a service user. We are reasonably comfortable with copying (or even addressing) letters to service users and also that some will make legal requests for their entire record, but how do we feel about full routine access to the live record? Technically, this is now possible. The new GP contract in England and Wales committed to all patients having online access to their full record by April 2020. Similar legislation has been passed in the United States. The pandemic has disrupted full implementation, but it seems to be coming, with medical defence organisations starting to prepare![11]

There are clear benefits to this with improved engagement and ownership by service users, but it will mean a change to the way clinicians work, The challenge is whether we will retrench and become more defensive, or be empowered and encourage this more. There are also specific debates to be had in psychiatry, such as whether full access should be modified for some groups such as those under 18 or with an intellectual disability.

Just One Login Please! Single Sign-on (SSO)

How would it be if you used one set of programs for all your clinical work? Many clinicians access several systems and thankfully password-management systems can now help with automatic logging in. However, consider doing clinical work though the same system that you use for admin and office tasks. For many people, this is Microsoft Office and, with Microsoft now having contracts with the NHS in many parts of the UK, this seems here to stay.

The pandemic introduced many NHS staff to programs like Microsoft Teams. So far, most areas have not begun to link the Office suite to their clinical systems, but technically

---

‡‡‡ www.alcidion.com/products/miya-precision/

this is becoming possible. More complex programs within the Office suite, like Power BI, can be used to automatically route referrals to a group of clinicians for processing or to receive messages about clinical alerts. This is supported by an active programme within Microsoft to engage with the healthcare sector – which receives a large amount of central government funding.

Summary

Well-connected systems that safely and ethically share information have a lot of potential to improve care and safety. Due to systems having developed organically and over long periods of time, the reality today is more piecemeal. There are several current initiatives to develop and improve the situation; the main barriers are often managerial or ethical rather than technical. Increasingly, the focus is on moving data out of big silos like hospitals to places where it can be accessed (when appropriate) by others.

References

1. Donne, J. Meditation XVII. In: *Devotions upon Emergent Occasions*. 1624. Scotts Valley, CA: CreateSpace Independent Publishing Platform.

2. Caldicott, F. *To Share or Not to Share: The Information Governance Review*. Williams Lea for the Department of Health. 2013: 119. Available at: https://assets .publishing.service.gov.uk/government/up loads/system/uploads/attachment_ data/file/251750/9731-2901141-TSO-Caldicott-Government_Response_ ACCESSIBLE.PDF (accessed 20 June 2023).

3. Wachter, R. *Making IT Work: Harnessing the Power of Health Information Technology to Improve Care in England*. Department of Health and Social Care. 2016. Available at: www.gov.uk/government/publications/ using-information-technology-to-improve-the-nhs (accessed 20 June 2023).

4. Kirkham, E. J., Lawrie, S. M., Crompton, C. J. et al. Experience of clinical services shapes attitudes to mental health data sharing: findings from a UK-wide survey. *BMC Public Health*. 2022;22: 357.

5. Great North Care Record. Why we have moved away from permission to view in the Great North Care Record. 2019. Available at: www.greatnorthcarerecord.org.uk/why-we-have-moved-away-from-permission-to -view-in-the-great-north-care-record/ (accessed 20 June 2023).

6. Wachter, R. *The Digital Doctor*: McGraw-Hill Education. 2017. Online. Accessed 20 June 2023.

7. HIMSS. Interoperability in healthcare. n.d. Available at: www.himss.org/resources/ interoperability-healthcare (accessed 20 June 2023).

8. Sipherd, R. The third-leading cause of death in US most doctors don't want you to know about. *CNBC*, 28 February 2018. Available at: www.cnbc.com/2018/02/22/medical-errors-third-leading-cause-of-death-in-america.html (accessed 20 June 2023).

9. NHS England. Open API policy. n.d. Available at: www.england.nhs.uk/digital technology/connecteddigitalsystems/inter operability/open-api/ (accessed 20 June 2023).

10. NHS England. What are integrated care systems? n.d. Available at: www .england.nhs.uk/integratedcare/what-is-integrated-care/ (accessed 20 June 2023).

11 MDDUS. Are you ready for online patient access to medical records? 28 February 2020. Available at: www .mddus.com/resources/resource-library/ risk-alerts/2020/february/are-you-ready-for-online-patient-access-to-medical-records (accessed 20 June 2023).

Digital Wellbeing
Using Technology Well

Toral Thomas and Paul Bradley

Digital should not replace paper – it should re-imagine it!
Professor Julia Adler-Milstein, 2018[1]

Technology as a Cause of Burnout or an Enabler for Better Health and of Wellness

Technology can both distress and impress us. It has become ubiquitous and for most people an intrinsic part of their lives. It is rare for most people to leave the house without a smartphone, for example. But pause for a moment and think about how you would feel if you looked at your mobile phone right now and saw the battery life was at 1%. Or if you could not find your phone at all? In just a couple of decades electronic communications, mobile phones and other smart devices have gone from being luxuries to an essential part of our everyday lives. On the one hand, a smartphone can replace multiple devices, improving portability and allowing end-user customisation, but that same range of features builds a dependence which can be challenging for many to manage.

Many proposed solutions for digital wellness rely on setting limits on our use of technology. However, when we return to our devices, systems or networks, we find others have not taken the same break that we have and now we have even more to deal with, engendering a fear of missing out (FOMO). A typical example of this is a clinician's email inbox, filled when they return from their holiday despite having an out-of-office reply in place. From copy-paste to reply-all emails, digital makes creating and sharing information almost *too* easy. Setting limits may temporarily manage the symptoms but fails to address the cause of the distress. A similar transition from the focus of healthcare from treating illness to enhancing wellness is needed for our approach to technology.

With many competing pressures, wellbeing can be an add-on when it comes to digital products. An argument could be made that user experience should be the priority as it is so critical to ensuring the success of digital healthcare. The 2017 Mental Health Atlas found that globally there is one psychiatrist and only 0.25 occupational therapists across most income groups per 100,000 of the population.[2] With the widening workforce crises across mental health globally and increasing clinician burnout in the face of a global pandemic it is more important than ever that digital enhances our wellbeing. This cannot happen if digital processes simply replicate paper ones.

Smartphones have been used to begin to reimagine healthcare. Examples of this include using apps for mindfulness; video calls with hospital specialists; viewing your medical record online and ordering medication to be delivered to your local pharmacy. The ability to empower citizens to manage their health through virtual health assistants or ambient monitoring technology has become science fact not science fiction.

Harnessing digital more widely in healthcare means transforming it but progress can be made by having a digital process replace or improve multiple paper or manual processes. This can include robotic process automation freeing us up to do clinical work by using natural language processing to code diagnoses and treatment. However, an internet search for the phrase 'clinician burnout' will bring up multiple articles on the electronic patient record. Atul Gawande's reflections on clinicians and their computers in the United States makes for sobering reading.[3] As clinical staff are asked to increasingly undertake administrative tasks as opposed to direct patient care, their career satisfaction decreases and their risk of burnout increases.[4] For true citizen and clinician engagement, wellbeing should be a focus at the start of any digital change and must remain at the heart of it.

We can promote wellbeing in digital by engaging with it, using digital to improve upon paper processes and always keeping our knowledge of digital systems current with regular training. It is not enough to treat the symptoms of anxiety and burnout when it comes to digital. It is better to not only prevent them, but to actively promote wellness instead. The rest of this chapter details some of the research behind this and practical steps you can take. Digital must be evidence based and appropriately tested but we must also evolve our idea of what evidence we use. Look to podcasts, blogs and other media and evaluate the ideas shared for yourself. Digital change is rapid change. We need to adapt to keep us and our patients from being left behind. If we engage effectively with digital transformation, we can get amazing outcomes for our patients and ourselves.

This chapter will look in more detail at some of the emerging challenges digital brings to our wellbeing. Practical solutions to address the causes of burnout rather than the symptoms will be the focus. Digital research is constantly evolving and by the time a paper is published there can already be new evidence available. A digital product can have evolved over several lifecycles into something completely different by the time the evaluation of the original product is complete. We live in an unprecedented time for creating data. The challenge is using this data proactively to improve quality and safety whilst reducing the burden on us all.

Why Care about Digital Distress?

The distress which digital systems in health cause is not trivial, leading to safety concerns and major issues in the workforce, often considered under the term 'burnout'. Burnout is formally described as a state of constant exhaustion, usually relating to work stress.[5] The impact of burnout on the medical profession in particular is a global crisis,[6] which has not spared mental health services. In some studies it has been found to affect more than half of all psychiatrists worldwide.[7-9] Digital tools are often cited as a cause, and you can see the face validity of this by looking at the faces of your colleagues when someone mentions a new digital system. One approach to preventing burnout is to enhance staff engagement and 'Joy in Work'.[10] Pause for a moment and think about this. Do you feel joy when you think about your work? If you do – what aspects enhance that joy and what aspects wear it down? Where did technology feature in your reflections?

The most widely used models of burnout consist of three factors: 'depersonalization, exhaustion and a decreased sense of effectiveness' (p. 898).[11] Focusing only on the exhaustion domain, 80% of doctors and medical students in the UK have been found to have high or very high risk of burnout in a large online survey.[12] In the United States, studies have consistently demonstrated high rates of burnout,[13,14] citing Electronic Health Records (EHRs) and electronic prescribing as major contributors.[15] The focus on records for compliance and billing contributes to a particularly high impact due to the requirement to make records which are not meaningful for the clinicians.[16] Automated notifications have also been associated with increased burnout.

The NHS Long Term Plan emphasises the role of digital technology as an enabler in the future of healthcare and in making the NHS 'a more satisfying place ... to work' (p. 94),[17] but mentions technology as a negative contributor to wellbeing. This approach reinforces the concept that digital cannot alleviate burden if people feel it is done to them rather than developed with them. Any digital innovation is likely to suffer from non-adoption or abandonment without considering its effects on the people using it.[18]

The NHS Staff and Learners' Mental Wellbeing Commission report from February 2019 looks at technology as being both a cause for and a solution to mental distress.[19] However, except for 'exploring' the use of technology to connect remote staff, the report does not explore technology and distress in any further detail. A review of trainee and trainer morale in the annual surveys from Health Education England focuses on issues like workload and supervision.[20] Technology can be a major cause of increased workload through numerous systems that do not communicate with each other (such as a prescribing system and a patient record) or having to log in to dozens of systems to carry out simple tasks. It can also alleviate burden by enabling remote teaching through social media journal clubs or virtual reality laboratories.

These issues are not restricted to the United States and UK. A Global Health Observatory report noted a 46% global increase in the use of electronic health systems.[21] In higher-income countries, more than 50% used digital systems in healthcare compared to 15–30% in low- and middle-income countries, respectively, but as these systems become more ubiquitous in health settings so too does their impact.

A systematic review and meta-analysis reports that burnout 'frequently associates with poor quality of care' (p. 555) with the caveat of publication bias.[22] Despite limitations such as the heterogeneity of burnout definitions in over 120 analysed publications, there is increasing evidence that there is an association between burnout and poorer quality of care.

Are We Always Anxious?

As we look to digital to ease our work it can instead be a source of increasing complexity, frustration and anxiety. As more records become digital, staff are spending more time entering data than engaging with their patients. A typical assessment appointment may last an hour but give rise to two or three hours of administrative tasks undertaken by the clinician. A group of mental health Chief Clinical Information Officers in the United Kingdom speak of 'DataMHageddon'– the potential for the collapse of healthcare because of the increasing burden of data collection on healthcare staff.[23] NHS sickness data from August 2020 indicates a sickness rate of 3.9%.[24] Despite the Covid-19 pandemic the most common causes cited are anxiety, depression and other psychiatric illnesses. Almost half a million days of work were lost as a result.

Anxiety disorders have been described in the literature for over 400 years,[25] and they affect around one-third of us during our lifetimes. From podcasts to open access journals there is now an almost constant barrage of information which our brains are incapable of absorbing. As information becomes always accessible, people are too. Clinicians can be praised as supportive and dedicated if they are always willing to answer a phone call or an email, regardless of the day or hour, but this constant level of alert takes a toll. What is your first thought when you hear a ringtone or notification from your phone?

With the developments in technology, perhaps it is inevitable that illness will follow. There is a strong correlation with anxiety and social media in young women,[26] and there is an ongoing debate between scientists around the role of technology on mental health in adolescents.[27] Woman are reported to have more depression and anxiety disorders then men do and there are many theories about this, including the way men and women access health services. The rise of depression and anxiety is a complex issue made even more challenging by the various instabilities in the world today, including financial insecurity, a global pandemic, and the ability of social media to spread both positive information and disinformation.

Many antidotes to modern life seem to focus on regression. We are often told to turn our phones off, create technology-free spaces and spend time away from our technology. This cannot truly alleviate the anxiety that the volumes of information and expectation overload creates. Distraction and time-outs do not deal with the fundamental problem. If we keep using digital in the same way that we use paper it can never enhance our lives or those of our patients. Digital must transform culture and enable new processes that focus on the person not the technology. It needs to be the best supporting player in our work – enabling but invisible. This means challenging people to practise in completely new ways. One example of this is the rise of dictation (human or artificial) in the background of a clinical consultation. The more data is required from clinicians, the more inventive we need to become to provide it.

The Rise of Social Media and Our Fears of Missing Out

No chapter on digital wellbeing would be complete without addressing the juggernaut of social media. From the early days of MySpace and Twitter to Instagram and TikTok, the reach and influence of social media cannot be denied. If we want to engage our service users and our future workforce, it is clear that we must engage in some way with social media. However, one of the many prices paid for increased connectivity is how amplified the consequences of our actions can become. A misplaced comment in person can cause momentary embarrassment, but an ill-timed Tweet or post can lead to death threats and the loss of a career. The world is getting smaller as our digital reach gets longer, bringing envy of lives lived on social media. If ignorance is bliss, then Instagram is insecurity.

The fear of missing out (FOMO) was first explored in the literature almost a decade ago.[28] Being connected helps us see what is out there and can inspire change, global movements and even revolution, but if we constantly wonder about the next great thing we can never truly live in the moment and enjoy what we have. Paul Dolan in his book *Happiness by Design* suggests that the things we choose to pay attention to define our happiness.[29] By this logic, if we spend our time constantly scrolling, we never focus on any one thing and will always be chasing happiness.

Positive initiatives have arisen through social media, including '15 seconds 30 minutes', using quality improvement (QI) methodology to improve the experience of work.[30] The concept is to take 15 seconds to do something that can save a colleague half an hour in the future. Other movements facilitated by social media include improving civility at work[31] and introducing ourselves to our patients with the simple phrase 'Hello, My Name Is . . .'.[32]

The key part of this social activism is that information was shared to allow people to act together. Media in isolation simply fosters more isolation. Using social media as a way of sharing our interests or finding new ones can be healthy when done in moderation. It is important to remember that with social media we are the product. Allowing social media platforms to guide our content choices can make us forget that we are ultimately in control. If we constantly wonder about the next great thing we can never truly live in the moment and enjoy what we have. One way to start taking control of your social media is to examine your feeds. The people and topics you follow say a lot about what you find important. The data we consume is as important to our health as the food we eat. By curating our social media more rigorously we can keep our minds a healthier space to inhabit.

The Discomfort of Going Digital

Change can bring anxiety and managing this anxiety is a large part of making a digital project a success. When we look at successful transformations there are almost always a few constant enthusiasts who drive the change and contain the fears of other colleagues. However, with high staff turnover, the team that started a digital project may not be the team that completes it and the enthusiasm can be lost. This can cause delays or even derail a project completely so the potential benefits are never realised.

Clinical engagement (or more specifically the lack of it) is a critical issue when it comes to change with digital. Using the Pareto principle, 80% of the concern may come from around 20% of your users. Perspective is key here and focusing on the early adopters may help create enough momentum to bring the laggards and sceptics along.[33] This will especially be the case if the benefits to service users and staff can be spelled out clearly, early and repeatedly.

The global coronavirus pandemic saw a sudden and sometimes dramatic uptake of digital tools by necessity. Concepts such as patient-initiated follow-up and reducing our carbon footprint had been discussed for some time. Suddenly healthcare systems around the world scrambled to provide digital alternatives to face-to-face care which had continued as the norm in most regions. The transformation varied from innovative ways of conducting eye examinations remotely to the more mundane video call appointments. If you pause to reflect, the idea of someone driving into hospital to discuss results of routine tests with a hospital specialist seems nonsensical now when this conversation could be held by telephone or video call. Resistance to changing practice had been maintained by a variety of factors, including financial; the payment to a hospital for providing a face-to-face consultation far exceeded the payment for providing a remote consultation.

It is impossible to consider digital wellbeing without thinking about digital inclusion and exclusion. For our patients to embrace digital (as we have with booking flights or shopping) it must be easy to use, convenient and, crucially, accessible. If your website is confusing and overloaded, it will add to patient anxiety in a time of crisis rather than smoothing access. Digital systems can work 24 hours a day, 7 days a week without any additional cost, making virtual therapy options markedly more convenient than those constrained to a particular time and day each week. From chatbots to user-centred design to influencing stakeholders to fund training and access (such as virtual consultation hubs at GP practices), digital wellbeing needs a whole-systems approach to work, acknowledging that even with the best intentions and design it is not for everyone. There will always be people and situations for which digital systems are not suitable, so alternatives must always be prominently presented. Choice is vital.

It is also important to avoid the fallacy of sunken costs; the notion that once time and resource has been invested in a project to deliver a new digital system, it must be seen through to completion. Some projects are just not viable, but their imposition can have both immediate negative effects and undermine trust in any future digital systems. Organisations need the courage to halt projects rather than foisting changes on clinicians. When mistakes happen (and they will) it is important to be clear, take responsibility and address it. Reflective practice can be really helpful, but avoid dwelling on what could have been; or 'if it's not going to matter in five years, don't spend more than five minutes being upset by it'.[34]

Digital without the Despair

Now we have seen what digital transformation should not be, we can consider a few aspects of how it should be. Before beginning any digital project, the leads need to think about how it will enhance whatever is being replaced. In many cases, this may mean an improvement in quality and safety but an increase in time. If this is the case, it is important to be transparent about this from the start and explain why the increased quality or safety makes the new process of benefit overall.

Digital gives a chance to reimagine work. Using simple, free online tools you can start mapping current processes and then explore how digital can simplify, enhance or entirely transform them. Getting patients and clinical staff involved early is key as the mapping will rely heavily on their input. It is also an opportunity to start the change management that is an inevitable part of any transformation. Some of these agendas will be explicit such as reassurance that a patient can still see a care professional when they need to. Other agendas will be more subtle and can include the fear of technology itself or that it will lead to redundancy.

To have true patient and staff buy-in, there needs to be a clear narrative of benefit to all those using the system that is regularly and clearly communicated. Framing projects in this way can often help share the vision of why the digital system is being considered in the first place. A lot of this will depend on the culture of the organisation you work in. Using proxy measures for culture and digital maturity (such as an overall Care Quality Commission rating or a Digital Maturity Assessment level) can give you a rough idea of the challenges you may face.

Good training is key to building clinician satisfaction with digital systems.[35] Clinicians may struggle to see the benefits of learning to engage with electronic patient records if this is demonstrated to them as an administrative function rather than a clinical tool to enhance safe, high-quality care. It may seem incomprehensible that clinicians would seek further training when upgrading their smartphone but not do so for the digital tools they use daily. A common refrain is that our clinical tools need to be as intuitive as those we buy in our private lives. There is a strong argument for improving user interfaces and enhancing user-led design.

Another important issue to consider is diversity. From seatbelts to medication, many things we use today have been tested for men rather than women. In her book *Invisible Women: Exposing Data Bias in a World Designed for Men*,[36] author Caroline Criado Perez looks at how this affects everyday life and the knock-on effects as a result. In just one example from Sweden, the way roads were cleared disproportionately disadvantaged women who were more likely to use walkways and public transportation and therefore were more likely to slip as these areas had not been cleared. This resulted in more injuries for women with more serious injuries and more hospital visits. From gaming headsets to phone sizes, design favours men and this cannot be healthy, especially when designing for the whole workforce. Along with patient involvement and diversity, there are various ways to consider how people will use the new product. Considerations for people who have learning and communication needs, dyslexia, colour-blindness and more are so important to improve access and can be easily facilitated using modern systems. If done well, technology can improve inclusion by offering a flexibility that traditional services could not.

What Actually Works?

Joy in Work has been adopted as an approach to mental health workforce issues in the UK by the Royal College of Psychiatrists.[37] Despite the increasing use of digital in UK mental health services, we are many years behind our colleagues in the United States and primary care where electronic systems are well established and research on alleviating the negative impacts has progressed further. One study in the United States relating to Joy in Work looked at 23 high-performing general practices.[38] Given the premise of this chapter, it will come as no surprise to learn that these practices did best with high administrative support for clinicians, better verbal communication, non-physician scribing and co-location of teams. In other words, focusing on the person rather than the technology. Although this is one way to approach digital transformation it does not actually leverage the power that digital can bring.

Another study in primary care in the United States is the Healthy Work Place trial,[39] which found that improvements in quality and reduction in error rates lagged behind improvements in clinician satisfaction and reduced clinical burnout. In other words, to get the quality and safety improvements required burnout and satisfaction to be addressed first. This is an exciting way to look at research in this area as it suggests focusing attention on improving joy and satisfaction at work, rather than focusing on the end product of burnout.

Popular media is full of ideas for improving our wellbeing. Each new article recycles the same themes – set boundaries for yourself, spend time with people/nature and try to have time away from technology. Whilst a hike in nature or turning off your notifications will provide respite, these ideas do not deal with the underlying problem. If you work in an organisation where 'reply all' is commonplace, your email inbox will always be heaving. Addressing these issues needs to start from the core.

Digital Wellbeing in the Workplace

There are two key elements to reducing your digital distress at work:

1. Engagement – from national surveys and with the added pressure of a pandemic time is in shorter supply than ever. Investing some time in a digital project will lead to more work in the short term but can reap dividends with reduced workload or improved quality and safety in the longer term. The ideal project will manage all three.

2. Education – digital cannot be a one-time experience. Digital products evolve and new products are regularly brought to the market. Surgeons would never use new kit for an operation without familiarising themselves with it first. However, many clinicians still balk at the idea of attending training for clinical systems which can cause harm or benefit on a much wider scale.

Clinical engagement with digital projects is key to their success. There is no one solution here – but the Global Digital Health partnership in their international overview report on barriers and enablers provides an excellent summary.[40] In essence, clinical engagement must be sought from the outset, clinicians must have meaningful input and the process should be focused on clinical aspects rather than administrative ones. The report also showcases the importance of digital workflows enhancing the proportion of clinician time spent on patient care rather than reducing this.

An example of this is electronic prescribing and medicines administration (ePMA). Electronic prescribing can take more time than writing a paper prescription. However, the digital version is legible, always accessible, allows for decision support and can be easily monitored across sites by a pharmacist. The benefits of ePMA in terms of improving safety from medication-related errors made it a focus for the NHS. A challenge to this is the use of agency staff in the NHS. Using electronic systems usually requires training and access credentials which may not be available to temporary staff the first time they take a shift in a ward. As well as addressing the practical issues, defaulting to paper can be made less appealing by demonstrating the value that the electronic process brings.

Digital Wellbeing at Home

Tablets, smartphones, smart speakers, smart heating and lighting – the list of technology we may have in our homes keeps growing. If you start with the idea that technology should enhance your life rather than complicate it, you are on the first step to achieving a healthy equilibrium with technology. There are genuine health conditions associated with technology excess such as a gaming addiction. These illnesses need early recognition and treatment. Video games have been around since the 1950s, but gaming addiction only found its way into the international classifications of disease in 2018.

The key thing to remember is that any time away from digital does not stop it being an issue when you return to your phone or turn your Wi-Fi back on. You need to examine your relationship with digital in a brutally honest way. There are ways to measure your online activity using your devices and ways to use them to set limits for yourself. This should not take away from the benefits technology at home brings you from simpler shopping, entertainment and connecting with those you love.

A new complication in recent years is the blurring of the boundaries between home and work. Digital allows a lot of work, even clinical work, to be carried out from home. With the rise of video calls, it can be tempting to book meetings or consultations back-to-back, especially with longer and longer waiting lists. As we become better at recognising illness, we often need to manage this clinical disease burden with dwindling resources. With digital, stretching yourself can be easier than ever and booking in rest periods into our digital calendar is not a familiar feeling.

Rather than having a break from technology, it may be more sensible to consider how you want to engage with it. During th Covid-19 pandemic lockdowns, society saw an increase in online gambling and domestic violence. The same technology that lets you gamble can also provide you with information and resources to recognise and escape from an abusive environment.

Take Control: From Helplessness to Wellness!

Prevention

Across healthcare it is now well recognised that rather than treat symptoms it is better to prevent them or actively promote wellness instead. Over 10% of the gross domestic product of the UK is already spent on treating mental illness.[41] Trends suggest these increasing costs are unsustainable and healthcare costs are expected to double by 2050. Prevention does not just promote wellness; it can save money and resources too. For example, research into prevention in children and adolescents shows enormous financial returns on investment.[42] For every £1 spent on group cognitive behaviour therapy for depressive symptoms there is an estimated return of £32 in benefit.

For clinicians and patients, prevention is applicable to digital contexts too. By working with other stakeholders, such as local authorities and charities, you can impact patient lives in ways that support digital engagement. This can include providing low-cost kit to help someone access video consultations or funding internet access to reduce digital exclusion. Supporting patients with sensors and wearable technology can promote active self-management. Patients can become a vibrant peer-support network from the comfort of their homes.

One of the programmes to advance digital in the National Health Service was the now abandoned Global Digital Exemplar programme. Global Digital Exemplars and Digital Aspirants were expected to produce digital blueprints as part of their funding. Blueprints cannot, by themselves, help address resource and cultural issues in other organisations. By looking more closely at the challenges in other organisations (sometimes described as 'redprinting'[43]) you can try and mitigate problems before they arise. Try this for the next digital project you have in mind, however grand in scale. Talk to other organisations who have implemented the product and look at their clinical safety cases, hazard logs, checklists and workarounds. Could any of these issues crop up in your organisation? Would the solutions your peers tried work for you?

Reinvention/Redesign

For a digital process to succeed, it must be better than the paper or digital process it replaces. A new project is a wonderful opportunity to look at current processes with a fresh lens. Involving clinicians and patients early may help with engagement. A great way to get clinicians on board is to show the benefits realisation from the outset. This may mean streamlining a bulky process or making the new process more patient led. Any digital process or product needs to be tested, embedded and then scaled up. An evidence-based framework for doing this has been proposed.[18] The framework considers adoption in terms of systems. These include the staff, patients and carers using the product but also the organisation deploying it and wider system pressures including government directives.

For example, SNOMED-CT coding and electronic prescribing have both been identified nationally for implementation in UK healthcare with benefits including better information sharing, resource planning and improving patient safety. Diagnosis and prescribing are complex processes – but they do not need to be complicated. To get wider adoption there must be a value proposition that benefits staff and patients. An example of this might be the use of natural language processing to scour clinical entries and suggest codes to clinicians as they write their notes. Robotic process automation, used for years in the insurance industry, has the potential to automate mundane tasks and free up clinical time for patient care. Leveraging digital in this way optimises its use and makes adoption much more likely.

User-Centred Design

It can be very tempting to come to design meetings with the final product in mind. In some cases, this feels like good preparation and in others a way to 'just do it'. Some projects can go through entire teams before clinicians and patients are brought in at the end to test what is essentially the final version of the product to see if they can tolerate it.

But do not aim for 'tolerable' as your satisfaction measure – aim for 'liberating'. New digital processes need to free up clinicians and patients, not burden them further. If there is meaningful input so staff and patients can see their ideas being implemented, there is much more of a chance this process will be embedded and scalable. In mental health, interpretation is the way to collaborate with someone and express their thoughts and feelings in a framework that is meaningful to them. It relies to some extent on the clinician and the patient being curious – with neither being an expert but going on a journey together. This is also a great way to look at user-centred design. It is vital not to come to the digital team with a product in mind but rather with a question. Be curious and encourage the curiosity of others. The phrase 'the art of the possible' might be replaced with 'the vision of the impossible'. Something might not be possible right now, but it may be in the short to medium term with a little thinking through.

User-centred design also carries responsibilities. It is incredible that as of 2021 there was still no standardised admission, care plan or discharge process in mental health services. If we all hold tight to our preferred processes, we cannot enact meaningful change. Compromise with customisation may be a palatable alternative.

Leadership

When we discuss wellbeing, many factors come into play. Resilience and autonomy are just two factors associated with wellness. Healthy people cannot thrive in toxic organisations. Leadership may feel like something associated with seniority but every clinician and patient is a leader and has the ability to positively influence digital, their wellbeing and the health of others. One way to think of digital leadership is the coach and star player model. When someone is first appointed as a clinical lead for digital or Chief Clinical Information Officer in an organisation, the temptation to be the 'star player' and always have an answer can be overwhelming. With all the jargon in digital it can be quite easy, especially if you have gone on additional training, to feel like the expert in a room. True digital leadership develops this potential in those around you. If everyone in your organisation feels that digital is 'done' by a particular person or team, they will never fully appreciate the role they play in its success. By approaching situations as a coach and developing your team as coaches, they will eventually mature to inspire the next 'generation' of coaches and so on across the organisation.

Linked to this is the idea of 'imposter syndrome'. At its core, imposter syndrome refers to an individual feeling they do not deserve a position due to perceived lack of expertise. Although not a recognised diagnosis, it is popular in the media and the subject of an

> **Box 9.1** Top 10 digital wellbeing tips
>
> 1. Set clear boundaries for *why* you use technology – not just *how* and *when*.
> 2. Stay connected with people – people before technology!
> 3. Think about the person not the process – user-centred design.
> 4. Explore service users' perspectives – avoid assumptions.
> 5. Be kind to your digital calendar – book in breaks as well as meetings.
> 7. Consider mentalisation – see things from the perspectives of others.
> 8. Get involved – make the technology work for you by taking an active role.
> 9. Keep learning – systems evolve and the way we work with them should too.
> 10. Always consider digital exclusion/inclusion and diversity.
> 11. Use these free tools to assess your relationship with technology and manage it differently: https://experiments.withgoogle.com/collection/digitalwellbeing.

international systematic review.[44] This includes everyone from adolescents to senior leaders. The researchers found it was particularly prevalent in ethnic minorities but present across all levels of experience and age. Imposter syndrome is associated with anxiety, impaired job performance and burnout. There is now progress in professionalising the role of digital technologists and clinicians, including having professional bodies such as the Federation of Informatics Professionals (FedIP) and the Faculty of Clinical Informatics (FCI).

It is key to remember that improving the health of our patients is why we come to work each day. Framing our work in this way can remind us of what our priorities need to be when we look at digital and wellbeing. These wellbeing tips (Box 9.1) summarise this section of the chapter.

The Future of Wellbeing in a Post-Digital Age

Despite its challenges, it is generally accepted that digital technology is here to stay. The frontiers of medicine in our digital world are shifting at pace. As sensors and wearables become cheaper and more accurate, the possibility for proactive healthcare improves. Social media provides a unique way to gain insight into our patients and social media giants are looking at ways to monitor this data to allow for earlier interventions if someone is at risk of self-harm or suicide. Some predictions and case studies of how technology can help in mental health services can be seen in this recent report on the digital future of mental healthcare and its workforce.[45]

As technology becomes more embedded in our lives it needs to serve as an enabler rather than an additional burden. In a world of measuring, we need to separate the signal from the noise. As regional shared care records mature and as we get better at extracting data from our siloed systems, we will have an opportunity for preventative medicine and population health management on an unprecedented scale. To do this well, we need to bring our clinicians, patients and citizens along with us and that takes a significant amount of trust. Being clear about the benefits to all; being transparent about the challenges; and being flexible in providing support can all boost wellbeing and improve the chances of success.

Box 9.2 Key learning points

1. Digital should reimagine paper, not just replace it – we must consider *why* we engage with technology and the value it can bring.
2. Boundaries around technology – both physical and emotional – are more important than simply taking breaks from it.
3. Education should be continuous – as technology evolves so must we, in order to keep leveraging its benefits.
4. Social interactions remain key – technology will not replace the deeper connections we foster with others – society functions best when we are compassionate to each other and ourselves.

Ultimately, we are responsible for our wellbeing and this needs to be one of the first things we consider when we look at digital, not the last. The key learning points in Box 9.2 summarise this chapter.

References

1. Adler-Milstein, J. NHS Digital Academy. 2018. Residential lecture to the first cohort of the NHS Digital academy. Permission provided by personal correspondence.

2. World Health Organization. *Mental Health Atlas 2017*. Geneva: World Health Organization. 2018.

3. Gawande, A. Why doctors hate their computers. *The New Yorker Magazine*, 5 November 2018. Available at: www .newyorker.com/magazine/2018/11/12/ why-doctors-hate-their-computers (accessed 23 June 2023).

4. Rao, S. K., Kimball, A. B., Lehrhoff, S. R. et al. The impact of administrative burden on academic physicians: results of a hospital-wide physician survey. *Acad. Med.* 2017;92: 237–43.

5. Freudenberger, H. J. Staff burn-out. *J. Soc. Issues.* 1974;30: 159–65.

6. The Lancet. Physician burnout: a global crisis. *Lancet.* 2019;394: 93.

7. Summers, R. F., Gorrindo, T., Hwang, S., Aggarwal, R., Guille, C. Well-being, burnout, and depression among North American psychiatrists: the state of our profession. *Am. J. Psychiatry.* 2020;177: 955–64.

8. Nuss, P., Tessier, C., Masson, M. et al. Factors associated with a higher score of burnout in a population of 860 French psychiatrists. *Front. Psychiatry.* 2020;11: 1.

9. Sarma, P. G. Burnout in Indian psychiatrists. *Indian J. Psychol. Med.* 2018;40: 156–60.

10. Perlo, J., Balik, B., Swenson, S. et al. IHI framework for improving joy in work. *IHI White Pap.* 2017;42: 8–21.

11. Summers, R. F. The elephant in the room: what burnout is and what it is not. *Am. J. Psychiatry.* 2020;177: 898–9.

12. Bhugra, D., Sauerteig, S. O., Bland, D. et al. A descriptive study of mental health and wellbeing of doctors and medical students in the UK. *Int. Rev. Psychiatry.* 2019;31: 563–8.

13. Shanafelt, T. D., West, C. P., Sinsky, C. et al. Changes in burnout and satisfaction with work-life integration in physicians and the general US working population between 2011 and 2017. *Mayo Clin. Proc.* 2019;94: 1681–94.

14. Locke, T. Medscape Global physicians' burnout and lifestyle comparisons. *Medscape.* 2019. Available at: www .medscape.com/slideshow/2019-global-

burnout-comparison-6011180%233 (accessed 12 December 2020).

15. Shanafelt, T. D., Dyrbye, L. N., Sinsky, C. et al. Relationship between clerical burden and characteristics of the electronic environment with physician burnout and professional satisfaction. *Mayo Clin. Proc.* 2016;91: 836–48.

16. Downing, N. L., Bates, D. W., Longhurst, C. A. Physician burnout in the electronic health record era: are we ignoring the real cause? *Ann. Intern. Med.* 2018;169(1): 50–1. https://doi.org/7326/M 18-0139.

17. NHS England. *The NHS Long Term Plan.* 2019. Available at: www .longtermplan.nhs.uk/ (accessed 23 June 2023).

18. Greenhalgh, T., Wherton, J., Papoutsi, C. et al. Beyond adoption: a new framework for theorizing and evaluating nonadoption, abandonment, and challenges to the scale-up, spread, and sustainability of health and care technologies. *J. Med. Internet. Res.* 2017;19(11): e367.

19. Health Education England. NHS Staff and Learners' Mental Wellbeing Commission. *Heal. Educ. Engl.* 2019; 1–96. Available at: www.hee.nhs.uk/our-work/mental-wellbeing-report (accessed 23 June 2023).

20. Health Education England. The National Education and Training Survey. 2020. Available at: www.hee.nhs.uk/our-work/ quality/national-education-training-survey (accessed 28 March 2021).

21. World Health Organization. Electronic health records. 2016. Available at: www .who.int/gho/goe/electronic%5Fhealth%5F records/en/ (accessed 30 March 2021).

22. Tawfik, D. S., Scheid, A., Profit, J. et al. Evidence relating health care provider burnout and quality of care a systematic review and meta-analysis. *Ann. Intern. Med.* 2019;171: 555–67.

23. Lovell, M. Chief Clinical Information Officer discussion group. 2019.

24. NHS Digital. NHS sickness absence rates August 2020. 2020. Available at: https:// digital.nhs.uk/data-and-information/publi

cations/statistical/nhs-sickness-absence-rates/august-2020 (accessed: 23 March 2021).

25. Bandelow, B., Michaelis, S. Epidemiology of anxiety disorders in the 21st century. *Dialogues Clin. Neurosci.* 2015;17: 327–35.

26. Haidt, J., Twenge, J. Is there an increase in adolescent mood disorders, self-harm, and suicide since 2010 in the USA and UK? A review. 2021. Available at: https://docs .google.com/document/d/1diMvsMeRphU H7E6D1d%5FJ7R6WbDdgnzFHDHPx9H XzR5o/edit (accessed 22 March 2021).

27. Haidt, J., Allen, N. Scrutinizing the effects of digital technology on mental health. *Nature.* 2020;578: 226–7.

28. Przybylski, A. K., Murayama, K., Dehaan, C. R., Gladwell, V. Motivational, emotional, and behavioral correlates of fear of missing out. *Comput. Human Behav.* 2013;29: 1841–8.

29. Dolan, P. *Happiness by Design: Finding Pleasure and Purpose in Everyday Life.* London: Penguin. 2014.

30. Pilling, R., Wadsworth, D. Creating joy in work is the only way to save the NHS. *BMJ Opin.* 2018. Available at: https://blogs .bmj.com/bmj/2018/10/12/creating-joy-in-work-is-the-only-way-to-save-the-nhs/ (accessed 21 December 2020).

31. Civility Saves Lives. n.d. Available at: www .civilitysaveslives.com/ (accessed 28 March 2021).

32. Granger, K. Hello My Name Is: a campaign for more compassionate care. *Hellomynameis.Org.Uk.* 2013. Available at: www.hellomynameis.org.uk/ (accessed 28 March 2021).

33. B2U. Crossing the chasm in technology adoption life cycle. 2020. Available at: www .business-to-you.com/crossing-the-chasm-technology-adoption-life-cycle/ (accessed 23 March 2021).

34. Hammond, R. 'If it's not going to matter in 5 years. . .' *Nursing Times*, 24 October 2017. Available at: www.nursingtimes.net/ students/if-its-not-going-to-matter-in-5-y ears-24-10-2017/ (accessed: 23 March 2021).

35. Longhurst, C. A., Davis, T., Maneker, A. et al. Local investment in training drives electronic health record user satisfaction. *Appl. Clin. Inform.* 2019;10: 331–5.

36. Criado-Perez, C. *Invisible Women: Exposing Data Bias in a World Designed for Men.* London: Vintage Publishing. 2019.

37. RCPsych. *RCPsych Workforce Strategy 2020–2023.* 2020. Available at: www .rcpsych.ac.uk/docs/default-source/ improving-care/workforce/rcpsych-workforce-strategic-plan-2020-2023.pdf (accessed 20 September 2020).

38. Sinsky, C. A. Willard-Grace, R., Schutzbank, A. M. et al. In search of joy in practice: a report of 23 high-functioning primary care practices. *Ann. Fam. Med.* 2013;11: 272–8.

39. Linzer, M., Sinsky, C. A., Poplau, S. et al. Joy in medical practice: clinician satisfaction in the healthy work place trial. *Health Aff.* 2017;36: 1808–14.

40. Global Digital Health Partnership. *Clinical Engagement in Digital Health: An International Overview of Enablers and Barriers.* 2019. Available at: https://s3-ap-southeast-2.amazonaws.com/ehq-production-australia/53772b23aabfdac950 fe9e0e217592030439c3b2/documents/attac hments/000/102/275/original/GDHP%5F ClinConEngage%5F2.06.pdf (accessed 23 June 2023).

41. World Health Organization. *The Case for Investing in Public Health.* 2014. Available at https://apps.who.int/iris/handle/10665/ 170471 (accessed 20 June 2023).

42. Khan, L., Parsonage, M., Stubbs, J. Investing in children's mental health: a review of evidence on the costs and benefits of increased service provision. *Cent. Ment. Heal.* January 2015: 1–24. Available at: www.researchgate.net/ publication/308084274_Investing_in_chil dren's_mental_health_a_review_of_evi dence_on_the_costs_and_benefits_of_in creased_service_provision (accessed 23 June 2023).

43. Thomas, T. Difficult journeys to digital maturity: why learning what not to do with a redprint could be your best route to successful transformation. In *Healthcare Efficiency Through Technology.* Expo 2021.

44. Bravata, D. M., Watts, S. A., Keefer, A. L. et al. Prevalence, predictors, and treatment of impostor syndrome: a systematic review. *J. Gen. Intern. Med.* 2020;35: 1252–75.

45. Foley, T., Woollard, J. *The Digital Future of Mental Healthcare and Its Workforce: A Report on a Mental Health Stakeholder Engagement to Inform the Topol Review.* 2019. Available at https://topol.hee.nhs.uk /downloads/digital-future-of-mental-healthcare-report/ (accessed 23 June 2023).

Chapter 10

Conclusion

The Future of Mental Health

Rob Waller, Mark Lovell and Omer Moghraby

Think like a system, act like an entrepreneur.
Matthew Taylor, 2022[1]

The quote above is there because it encompasses many aspects of what it means to be a digital mental health service but, sadly, also some of the reasons why progress thus far has been patchy.* Many digital initiatives have an initial fizz of activity but then fizzle out as the focus inevitably moves to something else. The NHS and most healthcare systems are complex systems with feedback loops and built-in compensatory measures. These come into play to restore the status quo and slow down change. They are designed to be safe – but sometimes work too well.

Instead, Matthew Taylor advocates that to bring in lasting change we need to think like a system – which here means digitising *all* parts of the NHS, placing digital transformation as core to the business of delivering healthcare and having the right incentives built in. We also need to act like an entrepreneur – being flexible and continuously adjusting the system after feedback from users (staff and service users). This 'continuous quality improvement' is out of kilter with the current big-launch IT projects where a new Electronic Health Record (EHR) is sold as the solution to all our problems. It resonates with Bob Wachter's observation that 'going live with an eHealth system is only the beginning' (p. 4).[1]

There is an increasing imperative that we get this right. There are now good EPR systems available that will cover most of what we do – but of course secondary care psychiatry is only part of the picture. All of medicine is digitising and there is an increasing army of tech companies developing apps and related healthcare products. Patients expect digital services and assume that in a modern world, clinician A will know what clinician B knows and not want to repeat themselves. Governments want to be seen as leading digital nations and attracting digital talent. Moore's law, the doubling of computer speed every two years, continues to hold as we move into the realm of chips built on the nanometer, atomic or even quantum scale.

In this book we have celebrated huge leaps forward and changes that, without disruptive triggers like the Covid-19 pandemic, might have taken decades. Yet this still needs incentives, strategy, focus, rigor and, most importantly for this book, digital psychiatrists to clinically lead the way!

---

* This quote from Matthew Taylor is one he has used a number of times, but specifically was shared at the Rewired Conference on 16 March 2022 in London. He was the CEO of the NHS Confederation at the time and it is based on a lifetime of experience working in the government and public sectors.

Everyone Gets to Play

One of the more shameful things about progress thus far is that it has been patchy. The evidence *for* digital systems is now too strong to ignore. They may not be perfect but even basic functionality will prevent the catastrophic errors in care that we have seen arise from illegible handwriting and making notes available across the system can improve patient experience, reduce clinician burden and even prevent unnecessary admission (see Chapter 3 on electronic records for the references).

This patchy adoption is due to several factors – early leaders were rewarded as 'global digital exemplars' but this now needs to spread, some areas just didn't have the digital leaders, some were managed by local authorities who have been hit hardest by reduced cashflow and also put social work systems first. However, this now needs to change. A digital system rarely saves an organisation money. However, they do bring different *kinds* of saving – less time spent on duplicating information, less resource spent on moving around paper notes, less money spent on negligence claims from incorrectly read instructions. However, good technology still costs money and often involves costs related to staff time using and maintaining the system.

The other aspect of patchy access is the digital divide – where not everyone has access to digital services. This can be due to poverty or a more general lack of digital skills. This is not necessarily something for hospitals to fix as the issues are complex and rooted in our wider society. Likewise, it should not be a reason for *not* introducing digital solutions for those who *can* use them to bring much-needed efficiencies and capacity sparing. National data shows that the number of households without the Internet is decreasing over time and governments are increasingly making this part of their wider plans.[2] What we as clinicians can do is insist that there is always choice, always a non-digital alternative and continue to advocate for digital inclusion where we can.

Everyone Wants to Play

Healthcare is big business. The number of healthcare technology companies has grown exponentially, and any digital leader will receive occasional requests for 'an initial chat'. The reason for this is that there is a lot of money in healthcare – the 2021 figure for the US mental health tech sector alone was estimated at $5.5 billion![3]

For some in mental health services, this is reminiscent of the controversial relationship mental health has with Big Pharma and reminds us of discussions about whether we should meet with pharmaceutical representatives or not. You will be pleased to hear that we are not going to tackle that particular debate here, but it is worth remembering the ethical principles we had to learn. Health tech is a new area with a slowly growing evidence base, changing regulation and the lack of maturity we have come to expect.

One commonly asked question is why this can't be left up to our colleagues in the IT department, but the reality is that they will likely be focused on the purchase and delivery of a big EPR system and more general network support and the IT department simply won't be aware of what is on the horizon in our specialty or the particular challenges we face. Also, the networks needed to ensure genuine benefit at a regional level into social care, primary care and into service users' homes – these are things that clinicians engage best with and who often already have these links.

So it will likely be clinicians who see the gap in the market, are contacted by a start-up company with a new app or are shown the apps our service users are already using. Here, the parallels with pharmaceuticals are again relevant. We don't move everyone in our clinic onto the new medication, we remember that there is more than one product on the market. We also remember that they cost money and someone has to pay.

A cynic may say that psychiatric medications have not changed much in the last 20 years and though there is a degree of truth in this, no one challenges the dramatic changes that they brought about when first introduced 50 years ago. We have seen sanity restored, people rising up from their beds and a radical reshaping of the way mental healthcare is delivered. Will digital transformation do the same?

Play Requires Structure and Rules

This new playground, where everyone wants to play and everyone should be able to play, does need some boundaries. Digitally speaking, fences are easy to overcome and we have devoted an entire chapter (Chapter 8) to integration and interoperability. So, it is perhaps more helpful to ask, 'Where's the teacher?' Who is the playground supervisor to keep play going well; who will stop the bullies and make sure everyone can join in?

Some countries are currently developing legislation to protect people from online harms. However, what we already have in medicine is in many ways quite good. We have the General Medical Council (GMC) and similar national regulators and the GMC guidance on 'Good Medical Practice' still holds.[4] The principles of good medicine have not changed, even if its delivery has.

Notwithstanding, people (service users, managers, fellow clinicians) will want to know if a certain digital leader knows what they are talking about. Organisations such as the Faculty of Clinical Informatics (FCI) cover this interface,[†] with clear competencies for clinicians with significant involvement in digital work.

As well as bringing rigour to those currently in digital roles, we need to mainstream this for all. In the same way as you would not leave child protection matters solely to the child protection coordinator, we cannot leave digital transformation to the clinical informatician. All psychiatrists need to be competent in using EHRs and conducting video consultations – and Royal Colleges are beginning to build this into training. All managers, including clinical directors, need to know the pros and the cons of digital change. And you can be sure that our service users will keep us abreast of their digital expectations too. None of these people need to be members of the Faculty of Digital Informatics – they just live in a digital world.

How Do I Fit In?

In the Introduction, we asked how your average mental health clinician can fit in. This is not those with specific roles or titles or time in their job plan, but the everyday clinician who works increasingly with technology. This is especially relevant to those early on in their career who will see things continue to develop over the next 50 years. We devoted an entire chapter (Chapter 6) to developing specialist digital clinicians, but what does it look like for everyone else?

We included a list that is repeated below but expanded (the parts in *italics*) and we have followed this up with some more detail about what we mean by digital innovation.

*   Learn more about the area: most mental health conferences will have a digitally focused seminar or two. *There are also podcasts you can listen to such as Digital Health Today,[‡] or*

[†] Go to https://facultyofclinicalinformatics.org.uk/.
[‡] Go to https://digitalhealthtoday.com/podcasts/.

shared conferences between clinicians, NHS IT staff and tech companies which are usually free to clinicians. One UK example is HETT – Healthcare Excellence Through Technology.[§]

- Do a quality improvement or audit project that requires data to be pulled from an Electronic Health Record. *Traditionally, projects would have been notes reviews, but there is a vast amount of data available if you know how to get it. The local analytics team should be able to extract quite a bit for you, even if this is just to get the project started.*

- Speak to local academics who research big data and assist with a project. *Not all local academic units do this, but you can also link in with DataMind,[**] which is a UK-wide collaboration that also taps into international datasets.*

- Submit a 'challenge' to your local innovation team and see how they increasingly engage with technology firms for a solution. *See more about this below.*

- Have a coffee with the clinical lead for digital in your organisation – there will be one! *There is no national list of these but ask your local eHealth department which clinicians they work with often.*

- Try video consulting/tele-psychiatry – even if just a test call with a friend. Then try it in your job. *The national system in Scotland allows you to make a test call as well as having lots of relevant information for service users and clinicians who are using it for the first time.[††]*

- Talk to a colleague in social work or the third sector and explore how your digital record systems compare. *Our main tip here is to keep it positive – take a 'can do' approach rather than having a group moan!*

- Find a local debate on the ethics of artificial intelligence and go along. *Remember that debates are often organised by people or organisations that have a particular perspective on whether this is good or bad.*

- Monitor your screen time on your phone or computer and reflect on how this is affecting you. *Whilst phones are designed to keep you engaged with them, both Apple and Android operating systems now let you monitor and restrict this to some degree.*

- For members of the Royal College of Psychiatrists – join the Digital Special Interest Group.[‡‡] For members of other organisations, see if they have a similar group.

- Sign up as an associate member of the Faculty of Clinical Informatics[§§] – £31 to £51 depending on salary at 2022 prices.

Innovation as a Way Forward

One way that all mental health professionals can get involved in digital projects is through innovation. Briefly, innovation is the pathway in healthcare that aims to bring new solutions to problems that cannot be solved by usual processes. If you consider a long waiting list as an example, there are improvements that can be made by being more efficient, working with referrers and even employing more staff. However, you do get to the point of diminishing returns in efficiencies and staff increases are limited for a variety of reasons. Hence something more major needs to change and the solution is increasingly a digital one.

[§] Go to https://hettshow.co.uk/.
[**] Go to https://popdatasci.swan.ac.uk/centres-of-excellence/datamind/.
[††] Go to www.nearme.scot/make-a-test-call.
[‡‡] Go to www.rcpsych.ac.uk/members/special-interest-groups.
[§§] Go to https://facultyofclinicalinformatics.org.uk/payments.

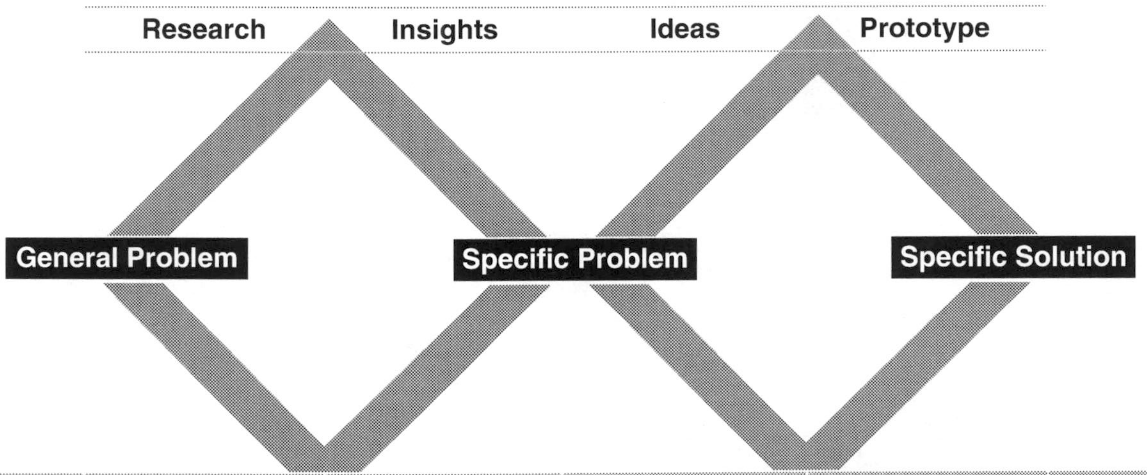

The Double Diamond labels:

Research — Insights — Ideas — Prototype

General Problem — Specific Problem — Specific Solution

Challenge	Discover	Define	Develop	Deliver	Implement
Identify the main pressures your service is under that cannot be solved by just working better or harder	Map current process and identify stakeholders. Share what has been tried already. Identify potential barriers to innovation	Bring clinical insights to insights from the 'Discover' phase to refine the general issue to a specific problem	Evaluate ideas as to whether they are workable or acceptable to staff. Work with service-user representatives on what is acceptable to them	Test out created solutions in small pilots, helping reject those that don't work and improving those that show promise	Starting with your current area, implement the solution and act as a champion or resource for other areas

Figure 10.1 The Double Diamond and how clinicians can contribute

Innovation typically starts with a challenge: 'to improve access and reduce waits', in this example. The problem is explored and then defined; then solutions are brainstormed, focused and then implemented. Examples in the area of waiting times might be using a screening questionnaire, offering patient-focused booking or offering an alternative treatment. Increasingly these will be digital solutions such as an online questionnaire or a website to pick an appointment or treatment through an app on your phone. The local health IT department and external technology companies are likely to be involved in the later phases of this but there are many roles for clinicians even if they don't feel they have specific digital skills.

Figure 10.1 illustrates this, following the 'Double Diamond' model for innovation,*** and shows how clinicians can contribute to each stage even if they have no particular knowledge of technology. Innovation challenges are usually prioritised by senior managers in line with organisational priorities, but anyone can suggest an area for consideration. Some areas have developed portals for any staff member to submit an idea for a challenge.†††

Summary

This book has taken you on a tour of digital mental health and told the story of both success and failure. However, the main messages are ones of opportunity and an imperative to change. Healthcare needs both digitisation (moving from paper to online) and digital transformation (doing things differently) to cope with the volume of information and the complexities of modern services. Service users will increasingly expect and even demand digital solutions. The main question we ask is whether clinicians will be at the heart of this change.

The answer, we believe, is a categorical 'Yes!' We have the clinical skills and experience that others simply do not. Now we need to have places at the table and a willingness to get involved at every level of change.

References

1. Wachter, R. M. *Making IT Work: Harnessing the Power of Health Information: Technology to Improve Care in England. Report of the National Advisory Group on Health Information Technology in England.* Department of Health. 2016. Available at: https://assets.publishing.service.gov.uk/government/uploads/system/uploads/attachment_data/file/550866/Wachter_Review_Accessible.pdf (accessed 27 June 2023).

2. Scottish Household Survey. 2019. Available at: www.gov.scot/publications/scottish-household-survey-2019-annual-report/pages/8/ (accessed 27 June 2023).

3. CB Insights. *State of Mental Health Tech 2021 Report.* 2022. Available at www.cbinsights.com/research/report/mental-health-tech-trends-2021/ (accessed 6 October 2022).

4. General Medical Council. Good medical practice. 2019. Available at: www.gmc-uk.org/ethical-guidance/ethical-guidance-for-doctors/good-medical-practice (accessed 27 June 2023).

*** This model was popularised by the Design Council in 2005 but has been widely adopted by healthcare innovation in the UK. Read more at https://en.wikipedia.org/wiki/Double_Diamond_(design_process_model).

††† See this example from Alder Hey Innovation in Liverpool, which also covers CAMHS innovation: www.alderheyinnovation.com/solutions-portal.

Appendix: Abbreviations

AI	Artificial Intelligence
cCBT	Computerised Cognitive Behaviour Therapy
DPIA	Data Protection Impact Assessment
ECT	Electroconvulsive Therapy
EHR/EPR/DHR	Electronic Health Record (other terms are Electronic Patient Record, Electronic Healthcare Record, Digital Health Record or Electronic Notes)
GDPR	General Data Protection Regulations
GMC	General Medical Council
GPS	Global Positioning System
IG	Information Governance
IT	Information Technology
ML	Machine Learning
NHS	National Health Service (also NHS England (NHSE) and Scotland and NHS Wales for those countries)
NHSX	A joint organisation across the NHS and the Department of Health and Social Care for digital, data and technology
NPfIT	National Programme for IT
PROMS/PREMS	Patient Reported Outcome/Experience Measures
PRSB	Professional Record Standards Body
RCPsych	Royal College of Psychiatrists
TEC	Technology-Enabled Care
VR	Virtual Reality

Index

Printed in the United States
by Baker & Taylor Publisher Services